BACKYARD

CHICKENS

Samantha Martines

Table Of Contents

INTRODUCTION

1 GENERAL NOTIONS ABOUT POULTRY — 5

2 DESIGNING CHICKEN COOP AND RUN PLAN — 17

3 WHY RAISE CHICKENS? — 33

4 CHICKS NURSERY — 47

5 FEED, WATER, AND TREATS — 67

6 PROS AND CONS OF RAISING CHICKENS — 81

7 GATHERING EGGS — 103

8 GETTING TO KNOW YOUR HENS — 113

9 LANDSCAPE GARDENING WITH CHICKENS — 127

10 PET THERAPY — 145

INTRODUCTION

Agriculture has become very relevant in society as it plays a significant role in the lives of humans. This implies that most life sustenance, including feeding, shelter, and clothing, is sourced from agriculture.

While there are various branches of agriculture, an exciting part that arouses the interest of so many individuals is poultry farming. Poultry farming's success is mainly dependent on the expanse of knowledge an individual possesses about the trade. To ensure you succeed in poultry farming, it is necessary to have the basic information of what it entails and the business's technical know-how. This implies a comprehensive idea of the skills, relevant workforce, and the resources needed to make this a reality.

Interestingly, poultry farming is an arm of agriculture that records no waste. Asides from making money off the chicken sale, the produce of the chicken and its dung also can be used to generate money. This is why it is sacrosanct to get detailed information of what poultry farming entails to benefit immensely from this agricultural activity.

It is erroneous that poultry farming requires little or no effort. Unfortunately, many individuals who delve into poultry farming without a defined purpose end up in failure and find it difficult to ascertain the business failure's cause. It is simply not enough to have the passion for poultry farming because when the desire is absent of commensurate action, it is as good as not attempting.

Poultry farming is an exciting venture if you own the nitty-gritty of the trade. Like every other business venture, if the right amount of energy does not fuel the zeal, it becomes nothing.

There is too much false information that society has associated with poultry farming. In situations where an intending poultry farmer fails to get his facts right, such a person loses foresight of his business goals and takes uncalculated risks. Without a doubt, there are risks in every business venture, and the poultry business is not an exception. But, when the risks are taken void of due consideration and a well-thought-out plan, it causes an unexpected disaster in the business activity.

Thus, there needs to be a solid foundation for its growth for poultry farming to turn out a success. The right atmosphere for poultry farming can trigger the right changes and cause a positive turn of business. As such, an intending poultry farmer needs to address specific aspects of the business. Considering that there are many breeds, it becomes pertinent to decide the correct species/breed to settle for and what such breed entails throughout its developmental phase.

It is certainly not going to be an easy task as it requires a lot of attention and dedication. With the right effort in place, there will be minimal or no losses during the business. In the course of the book, relevant and insightful information will be adequately discussed, which would guide individuals who are considering venturing into poultry farming. It also addresses all questions that come to the mind of budding poultry farming while also providing solutions to poultry problems and dispelling doubts from the heart of poultry farmers.

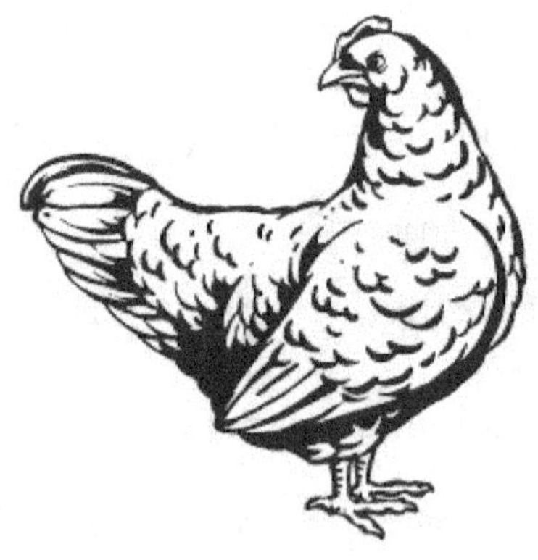

CHAPTER ONE
GENERAL NOTIONS
ABOUT POULTRY

Poultry farming, no doubt, is one of the most practiced aspects of agriculture. Therefore, it comes as no surprise that various individuals have a varying opinion of what they think about agricultural activity. There are so many misconceptions about what poultry farming should be. Ironically, most of these opinions and beliefs are hinged on personal or traditional reasons. Some of these opinions are fallacious and nowhere close to the truth of what poultry farming entails.

Legal rules for poultry

The importance of chicken and poultry farming in the United States cannot be overemphasized. To ensure that this agricultural activity is not abused or neglected by individuals, the United States federal government has put together legal acts to protect chickens and related activity. This does not hint that the government interferes in how chickens are bred or fed; they are only solely concerned about ensuring that things are done following the expected societal norms.

In the United States, chickens constitute a greater percentage of slaughtered animals every year for food and other purposes. This proves that chickens are greatly significant in the United States. To ensure that chicken and poultry farming is protected, the government of the US to set up the following acts:

The humane slaughter act: This act was set up to ensure that animals are not slaughtered in an inhumane way. Bearing in mind that specific individuals may be insensitive when snuffing the life out of animals, this law stipulates that before chickens or other livestock are slaughtered, they must be unconscious to make it less complicated to bear the pain. Thus, before killing or hoisting any animal, they should be given any form of a blow to the head. This would leave them unconscious and would make them not feel the full impact of the pain that would be unleashed on them. The United States federal government stipulates that this law be effectively carried in the slaughterhouses but excludes chicken and poultry. The only state in the US that emphasizes humane slaughter acts on broilers is Chicago.

The twenty-eight-hour law: The US government enacted this law to ensure that animals that are being transported are adequately treated. Thus, in transporting animals, it is expected that the animals that are transported do not exceed 28 hours without getting a minimum of five hours rest to be fed and watered. The law stipulates that the only exception to this rule is when the animals are transported in a spacious vehicle and gives them adequate room to rest. This law intends to control the large number of animal deaths that are recorded whenever they are transported. In 1994, this law was reenacted to address these animals' loading and unloading systems and ensure that their habitats were also rid of dirt.

Unfortunately, this law does not apply to chickens and poultry.

Misconceptions about poultry farming

There are some myths that individuals associate with poultry farming. Some of them are as such:

A chicken can lay as many eggs as possible in a day: This is a fat lie! As a matter of fact, a chicken can only lay one egg in a day. This is a result of the number of hours that are involved in egg formation. It takes about 25-26 hours for an egg to be formed. It is prevalent to see chickens lay eggs mainly in the morning and maybe a few in the afternoon or evening. It is fallacious to assume that a chicken can lay more than one egg in a day. It is not possible!

Broilers grow fast because they are fed with hormones:
This is nowhere close to the truth. A lot of people are always amazed at how big broilers grow in a brief period. Thus, they seem to attach all manner of conclusions to their thoughts in a bid to make sense of the broiler's development. The only factors responsible for broilers' rapid growth are proper management, genetics, housing, and nutrition. Poultry farming abhors the use of hormones in poultry as it is considered to be an illegal act.

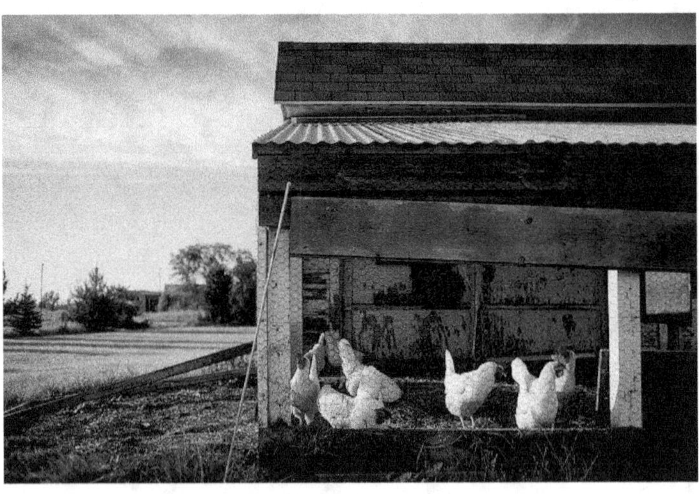

Yellow yolks are the most nutritious: It is difficult to ascertain how people came up with such conclusions and erroneous thoughts. The nutritional content of egg yolks is the same irrespective of the color of the egg yolk.

Cocks crow only in the mornings: Cocks crow to alert other chickens of impending danger or as a means of showing dominance, and this is possible at any time of the day. As such, it is not strange to see a cock crow either in the morning, afternoon, or evening. It all depends on the occasion that warrants such a response.

It is challenging to train chickens: Contrary to what many people think, chickens can be easily trained and regarded as a clever set of animals. It is difficult to hide something from a chicken because it would still uncover where it was hidden.

Chickens only eat vegetation: People believe that chickens can only feed on vegetation, but I'm afraid that's not right. Chickens do not just eat vegetation only but can also consume other types of foods.

There is no need to deworm chickens: This is where many people get it all wrong! Chickens are also susceptible to various diseases, and the only way to keep them safe is to ensure that they are adequately dewormed and accordingly. If this is done, it keeps them away from ailments such as tapeworms, roundworms, and other types of worms. More so, if chickens are not dewormed, it also affects their eggs.

Organic medication given to chickens is free from harm: Very false! While there are good organic medications that can be administered on chickens, some are detrimental to these chickens' health. Interestingly, modern medication is preferred and safer to be administered to chickens if used correctly than organic medication.

Chickens cannibalize each other if their bodies lack calcium: This is simply incredible! Chickens would always exhibit one form of unpleasant behavior or the other irrespective of how fed they are. These unwelcome behaviors are commonly referred to as vices. The best means of controlling such acts from chicken is to debeak or space them appropriately.

What to do and what not to do in poultry farming

Starting poultry farming requires a lot of conscious effort. That is, you must be adequately armed with the right attitude and discipline for the business. As a budding poultry farmer, what are those things that you must put in place before commencing with poultry farming? How do you go about them? Some of the basic requirements you need to attend to are:

Business plan: What structure do you want your poultry farming business to take up? What are your goals for venturing into poultry farming? A formal statement would help you define your goals and estimate how much is required in the course of the business.

An area of interest: There are various niches in poultry farming. You must identify the areas of poultry farming that arouses your interest the most and stick to it.

Location: Where do you want to situate your poultry farming business? What drives you the most about such an environment? You must secure a good location that is well-protected from theft and other social vices. In the same vein, get a good site that will help you minimize cost and reduce expenses that you are likely to incur on transportation.

Appropriate structure and feeding: You must give your poultry farm a good structure. There are various poultry structures. Ensure that you get one that you will be able to work with. Feeding is also a crucial aspect that you must consider. Therefore, get the appropriate feed for your chickens.

The don't's

Don't procrastinate: Nothing kills a business idea faster than procrastination. Always remember, if you can think about it, you can do it.

Don't settle for what you have no idea about: Just before deciding on any niche in poultry farming, ensure you have adequate information on what it entails. It would save you the cost of recording losses in the business.

CHAPTER TWO
DESIGNING CHICKEN COOP AND RUN PLAN

The chicken coop is also known as the henhouse. It is a place where you can securely chickens and other birds. The chicken coop also contains various nesting boxes that create space for the hens to lay their eggs. Also, it serves as a place where hens roost. To make chickens more comfortable in the coop, you may decide to add straws to it and make it easy for them to sit. The chicken coop's external environment possesses a fenced-in run that enables the chickens to make a run during the daytime and still stay away from danger.

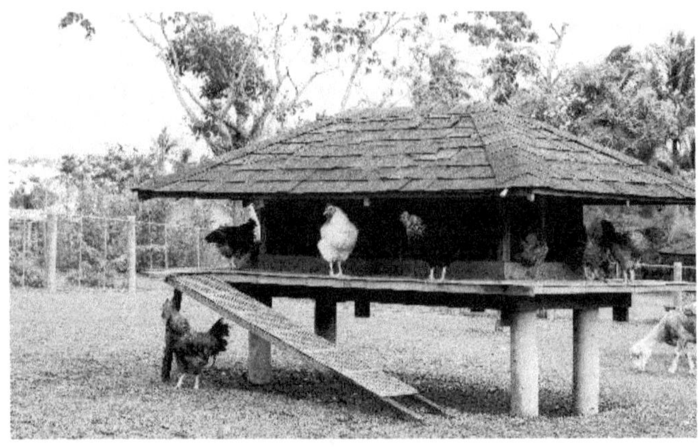

The importance of chicken coop cannot be overemphasized. It is no doubt that chickens are always easy prey for predators. Thus, the only way to keep them safe is to ensure that they are not within reach of predators. This is why it is necessary to get the right chicken coop ideas for your chickens. This would not only save your chickens from being attacked by stronger animals but would also save you the losses you are bound to incur when they are attacked.

For every budding poultry farmer, it is always a battle to ensure that the chickens are safe. While there are always many options to choose from, these options may not be suitable for you. The only way to make this possible is to survey the poultry farm's environment and identify the potential threats to your chickens' safety. If this is successfully carried out, there are higher chances that you would build the right chicken coop design to protect your chickens.

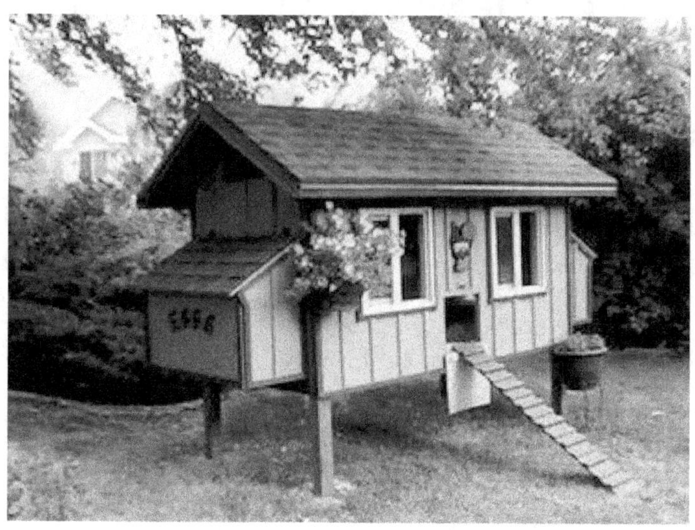

Some cozy chicken coop design ideas are:

Construct your chicken coop with stilts: In times past, generally, it was believed that chicken coop should be built with contact to the ground. Unfortunately, this exposed the chickens to a lot of dangers and threats. Thus, when it rains, the soil becomes damp, making it easy for termites and mot to invade your chicken coop, thereby making them prone to these unpleasant attacks. Also, this affects the well-being and development of the chickens and encourages the presence of predators. But, when the chicken coop is constructed with stilts, it takes the structure up into the air and avoids the rainy season's dampness. Interestingly, this makes it difficult for them to become prey to predators as no predator would find it easy to get a hold of chickens when they are far off the ground.

Proper lighting effects: Winter times are commonly associated with shorter days and bad light. In winter times, it is very common to notice a reduction in the egg production of chickens because of the poor lighting conditions. An excellent way of helping them maintain or improve their egg production is by illuminating the chicken coop's interior. This gives them the feeling that the days are longer and helps them stay productive during this period. All you need do is to find a healthy spot in the chicken coop and place the light source. With this, the interior of the chicken coop looks brighter.

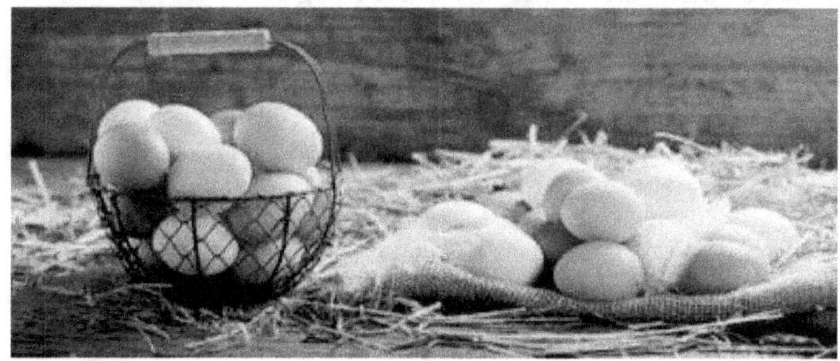

Encourage ventilation: Chickens also need appropriate ventilation. When the chicken coop is poorly ventilated, the chickens are exposed to illnesses that would affect their meat and egg production. So, to keep them active at all times, it is necessary to build a chicken coop with windows or other alternative means of ventilation. Another importance of having proper ventilation in the chicken coop is that it protects your chickens from being too hot when the weather is too hot. Asides from building your chicken coop with a window, an alternative means of encouraging ventilation are to let in the air into the cell through the roof of the coop. That is if the top of the chicken coop is slanted. When doing this, it is pertinent to get a chicken wire that can protect predators from coming into the coop while also enabling your chickens to receive proper ventilation.

Include a walk-in in your chicken coop: The idea of a walk-in is to save you the stress of always doing hectic cleaning that may leave your body feeling sore. Rather than favor an enclosed space that gives the chickens minimal entry and exit into the coop, it is best to have a walk-in, making it easy for the chickens to enter and leave the coop at any time. The ideal way to go about this type of chicken coop design is to ensure that the chicken coop has its latch, as this would keep the chickens secure in your absence.

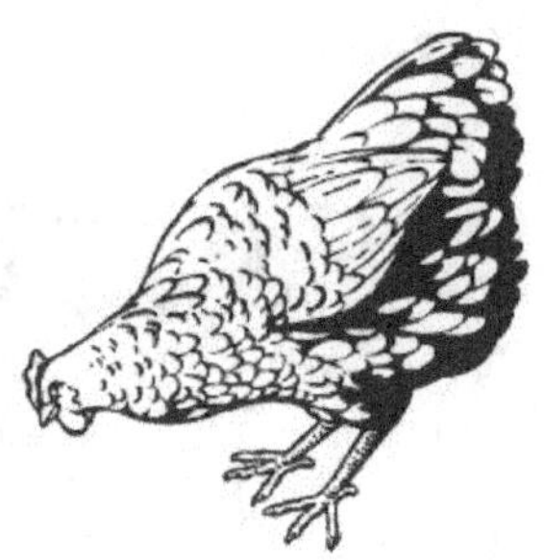

A mobile chicken coop: The idea behind this design is to enable ease of movement. Thus, if you do not have any particular location you want to build your chicken coop, the mobile chicken coop is the right choice for you. It protects your chickens from unfavorable weather conditions as you have the willpower to change the chicken coop's location whenever the need arises. One disadvantage of this design is that you would not be able to attach a run to it. But, it saves you the stress of worrying about your chickens' safety during unfavorable weather conditions as you are in the position to make healthy choices as it concerns your chickens.

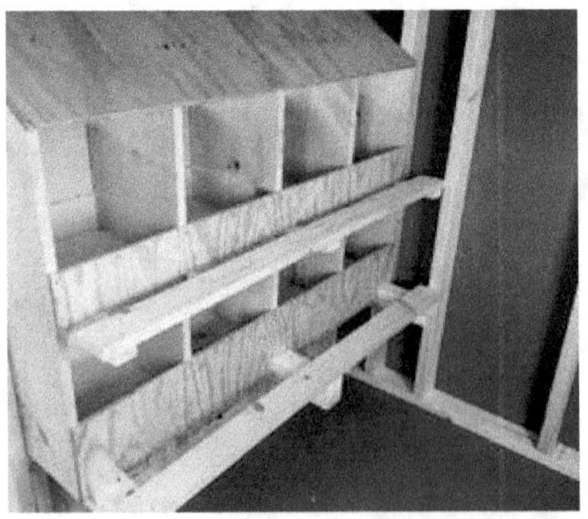

Make use of a rain collection system: It is always difficult to pass water into your chicken coop all by yourself. This is a lot easier when you have the right strategy in place to make the process faster. Interestingly, rainwater is safer than tap water. This is so as it contains no chemicals that may affect the lives or development of your chickens. So, with the rain-collection system, you depend on rainwater during the rainy season to give water to your chickens rather than manually.

The use of a shade: The use of shade for your chicken coop is crucial because it protects them from harsh weather conditions. Carefully constructing the chicken coop under a shade helps the chickens to stay cool during the summer period, and also, in winter, it helps them stay warm.

What is the ideal size of a chicken coop?

When considering your chicken coop size in poultry farming, you must bear in mind that several factors require your attention to this effect. Ironically, many people seem to believe that the chicken coop needs to be very big and spacious as this can make chickens feel very comfortable. Well, this is very far away from the truth. The only time a chicken coop needs to be very large is if the chickens in your poultry are in thousands of numbers.

Before making hasty decisions on how large the chicken coop should be, it is essential to answer some questions as they affect your choice of poultry farming. These questions are: Do you want your chickens to roam around freely? How many hours in a day do you intend to keep your chickens in the coop? What is the number of chickens you want to raise?

The above questions are a determinant factor in determining the size of your chicken coop. If you intend to keep chickens less than 10, you do not need above 18 square feet, and the run would also not exceed 90 square feet. The reality is that you do not need excessive space for your chicken coop.

All that you need is to ensure that the chickens are comfortable wherever you allocate to them. The ideal way of calculating how large your chicken coop needs to be is to realize that your chicken requires about 3 square feet per chicken. Thus, to get the right size of your chicken coop, multiple three (3) by the number of chickens you have, which would give you the right idea of how much space you need to get for your chicken coop.

The disadvantage of getting an extremely large chicken coop is that it makes it difficult for your chickens to generate the heat needed to keep them warm. When you have a large chicken coop with just a few chickens in the coop, this may likely bring about more harm than good. Nonetheless, if the chicken coop is not large enough, the chickens will pass across various types of diseases to one another. Just like every other pet, when your chickens are giving adequate room to spread their wings, they become less prone to diseases and make them feel comfortable.

Another factor that should be adequately considered is the resting space for the chickens. Your chickens require rest, especially at night. It is sacrosanct to get them the correct type of space that is essential for their proper rest. Although, it is no news that chickens huddle together, especially at night. While this is true, it is also suitable to provide them with the right type of space.

As a poultry farmer, it is your responsibility to decide where your chickens would roam. This decision is solely up to you. You can choose to create a run for your chickens or, better still, allow them to walk around your garden as they want. However, if you wish to make a run for your chickens, ensure that the run is portable because it will always be boggy during winter times, which would put you in a position of constantly changing your chicken's bedding.

Importance of a chicken coop

There is various importance associated with the use of chicken coop. They are:

It protects them from predators: The use of a chicken coop protects your chickens from predators. The dangers of exposing chickens to predators are that a single predator can affect the entirety of your flock. It is expected that you should lock up the chicken coop at night with the aid of a lock, and then during the day, you could leave them to have a run. But, the run of your chicken coop should have a fence that would protect them during the daytime.

It aids your garden's growth: When you leave your chickens to go for a run in your park, they are going to leave their droppings on your garden. The importance of their droppings in your garden is that it helps your garden blossom and grow beautifully.

Healthy eggs: With your chickens, you are confident of getting about one or two eggs in a day. Supposing you have several chickens, you may be fortunate to get as much as a dozen eggs every day. Also, you are confident that the eggs are always going to be fresh and better than the ones that are sold at the various local stores around you because you know when they were produced.

Keep the environment clean: Chickens are also instrumental in keeping the environment tidy and clean. This is because they would help you eat the weeds in your garden and ensure the place is free of weeds. Also, these chickens would help eat any fruit that falls off your trees or garden, which would prevent a situation where you have rotten fruits littered all over the environment.

Chickens are an excellent way to control bugs: Bugs are very destructive and can render your garden ugly. But, the spread of these termites can be controlled with the use of chickens. These chickens would help to prevent the spread of the termites by eating them up.

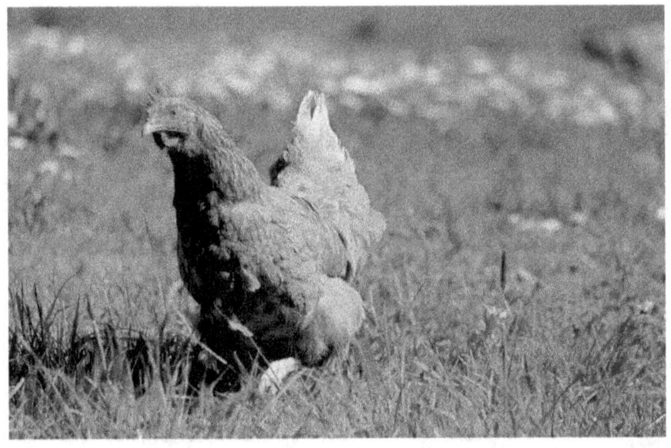

CHAPTER THREE
WHY RAISE CHICKENS?

Of course, there are pretty several agricultural activities you could venture it. So, why choose to raise chickens over the others? This is always a question a lot of individuals ask. Without a doubt, there are other agricultural activities that are more profitable than raising chickens. As such, any individual would always need an appropriate answer to the benefit of raising chickens offers than the other agricultural aspects cannot offer.

There are several reasons to raise chickens. So long as you have a place of your own, then you may just be able to raise chickens with less difficulty. Interestingly, raising chickens is less expensive, and it also gives you the benefits of feeding your family with good healthy proteins. Chickens, irrespective of breeds, can provide your family with abundant meat and egg. In raising chickens, you are also assured of making money in no difficult time. Unlike the other agricultural aspects that may take a longer time for you to make some profit, chickens enable you to make money off it by selling some of the eggs it produces. In the same vein, chicken droppings can also be used to fertilize your garden and can also be sold off to various individuals who require manure. So, virtually everything that has to do with chickens is profitable.

Mix flocks- Pros and Cons

Raising chickens of different flocks is always an interesting thing to do, but it requires a lot of conscious effort to make it come out successful. It would help if you were mindful of various factors when considering raising mixed flocks in your poultry farm. Some of these factors are:

Weather conditions: While you may nurture the thought of having various chicken breeds on your poultry farm, it is also necessary that you look out for weather conditions and how they may affect the chicken species. Thus, settle for chicken breeds that can tolerate both the hot and cold weather conditions.

Life spans: Certain chicken breeds can live for a longer time. It is expected that you favor such chicken breeds to reduce the losses you are bound to encounter.

The personality: The various chicken breeds have different personalities. While some chicken breeds are shy and quiet, others are very active. Before settling for chicken breeds, ensure that you pay attention to what works best for you and your family.

Colour and size of the egg: The egg's color and size are essential factors to consider when choosing a chicken breed. If you want an improved color and size of your chicken eggs, do adequate research before settling for any chicken breed.

Size of chickens: This is very important and should not be taken for granted. The size of your chicken determines how large the coop would be. So, if you want to get various chicken breeds, ensure that you have just the right amount of space to accommodate them to prevent the spread of diseases amongst them.

Pros and cons of a mixed flock

The pros

Some of the advantages of raising mix flocks are:

It makes it easy for you to identify the various breeds of chickens. Thus, if there is a situation where you need to find out what is happening with your chickens, the differences in their species make it easy for you. This is especially true when you have about two to three different breeds on your farm. You would be able to identify the differences between the chickens and know how best to care for them.

Also, it is easier to identify sick or injured chickens among your flocks. While this is true, it also makes it easy for you to appreciate the variations in the personality of the various breeds. With the different breeds, it is easy for you to identify the chickens that are ailing and administer the right treatment to them so that they do not affect the others

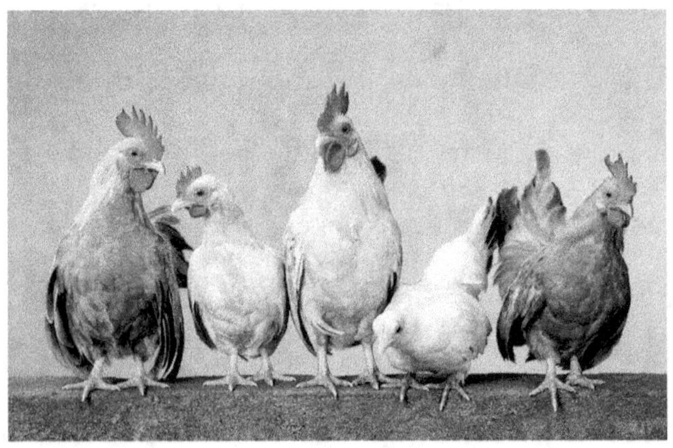

More so, as a result of the differences in the chicken breeds, it is easy to distinguish the chickens that are laying from others. This is because various chicken breeds produce eggs in different sizes and shapes. So, a glance at the eggs would aid you in understanding the productive chicken breeds. The colors of the various breeds vary. Some of them are white, olive, and dark brown, and bluish. With the proper sense of which chicken lays that, it is easy to identify the chicken breeds that lay an abnormal egg in the poultry farm.

Furthermore, with a mixed flock of the chicken breed, you are certain of getting an all-year-round egg production. It is no news that the various chicken breeds lay eggs at different times of the year.

While some of these breeds will comfortably lay eggs during the winter season, others may become active during the summer season. In all, as a poultry farmer, you are confident that you would indeed have a good production of egg all-year-round. With this egg production, you are also sure of getting other chicken breeds in the process. When various species mate and the hen lays an egg, there would be a mixture of both breeds to produce another breed.

Lastly, an advantage of mixed flocks of chicken breeds is that you would get a few broody chickens. As a poultry farmer, you may want to hatch some of the eggs rather than just sell or consume them. If this is it, then you require making use of a broody chicken. With a variety of chicken breeds on your poultry farm, you can get just the right type of chicken to help you hatch the egg.

Cons of mixed flocks

Some disadvantages of mix flocks of chicken breeds are:

Bullying: This is a common problem associated with having mixed flocks of chicken breeds on your poultry farm. While some chicken breeds get along easily, some do not. Chickens, in general, are territorial and can also be sometimes aggressive. The resultant effect of this is that some of the weaker chicken breeds may either die or get seriously injured by the stronger breeds.

The spread of diseases: As expected, keeping various chicken breeds together can lead to the spread of diseases from one to another. Also, some chicken breeds are susceptible to infections, and as such, they act as carriers and spread diseases amongst the others. It is easier to treat a particular disease outbreak in a chicken flock against a breed flock.

Poor nutrition: Contrary to the general belief of the concept of nutrition, poor nutrition is not necessarily being underweight or overweight. It is the state when the chickens are not fed with the appropriate nutrient contained in their food. Because of the differences in the breed of chickens, they will require special meals to suit their development. If all the breeds are fed with just one type of food, there are cases that their growth will be affected, and this can lead to the death of the chickens.

The wise selection of chicken breeds for eggs and meat

Many poultry farmers are constantly faced with the problem of the choice of chicken that should be on their poultry farm. Well, as a poultry farmer, your choice of a suitable chicken breed to keep on your farm depends on so many factors. These factors include your intent of raising the chickens, your budget, and available space. Nonetheless, a lot of poultry farmers raise chickens for the benefits of the eggs and meats they would get out of it.

While there are quite a handful of chicken breeds to choose from, it is necessary to make the proper research before settling for any type of chicken breed. While most chicken breeds lay eggs, the best type of chicken breed in the production of eggs is Rhode Islands, Sussex, and Plymouth Rocks. This is because these chicken breeds do not out on excessive weight as common with commercial chicken breeds. Also, these chicken breeds do not lay eggs as quickly as the commercial chicken breeds, but they certainly have a more productive life of laying eggs. Another chicken breed that lays good and large eggs is white leghorns. These chicken breeds are good, but they require a lot of food. Thus, before settling for these chicken breeds, it is necessary to understand their eating habits.

In addition, several other chicken breeds are also essential in the production of eggs. They are Australorp chicken breed, Lohmann brown classic chicken breed, Golden comet, Marans, La Bresse, and Hamburg. All of the aforementioned chicken breeds are good in the production of eggs.

In meat production, there are always certain chicken breeds that are very significant in this regard. Interestingly, some chicken breeds play dual functions such that they are good for meat production and are also significant in egg production. Some of the best chicken breeds for meat production are Cornish cross, Jersey Giant, Bresse chickens, Orpington, Freedom Rangers, and so on. These chicken breeds are good sources of meat production, and they also tend to feed well. But, it is important to understand that the various chicken breeds grow at a different rate. So, it is no surprise if a particular chicken breed is ready for consumption before another.

Where to buy chicks?

There are so many places to purchase chicken breeds, but it is safer to purchase chicken breeds from a reputable hatchery. A perfect place to buy chicken breeds is the NPIP. NPIP is an acronym for the National Poultry Improvement Plan. It is a system that hatcheries and poultry farmers can identify with. This body is charged with the responsibility of carrying out a check on all the birds and chickens in the poultry farms. It is a voluntary organization and does not in any way impose membership on poultry owners. However, there are some great benefits attached to hatcheries that identify with NPIP. One of such benefits includes the regular testing of chickens to ensure that they are rid of any form of disease or illness. As a matter of fact, quite a majority of large hatcheries identify with NPIP as a means of protecting the lives of their flocks as well as their investment.

When a poultry farmer refuses to identify with NPIP, it does not mean that such a farmer is at the risk of having sick flocks; it is only a means of playing safe. Therefore, it is advisable to buy chicken breeds from NPIP certified hatcheries. This is necessary to help address the issue of strange behavioral traits or diseases associated with the various chicken breeds. Nonetheless, it is strongly suggested that even after purchasing chicken breeds from NPIP, they should also be quarantined to prevent the outbreak of any unpleasant disease amongst your flocks.

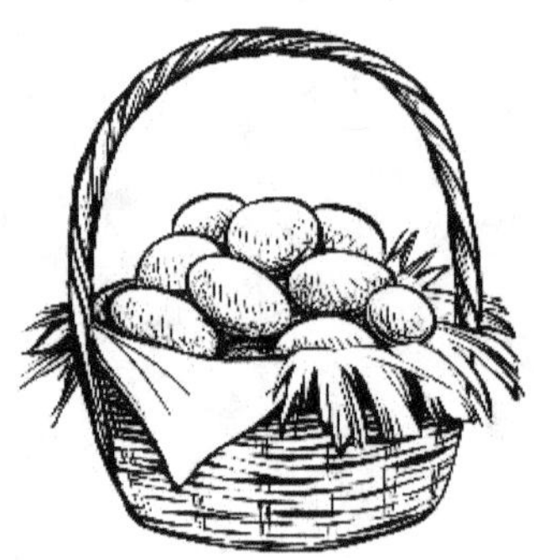

CHAPTER FOUR
CHICKS NURSERY

Baby chicks are an adorable and fascinating watch, especially as they try to get familiar with their environment. While this seems to be so much fun, there are lots of disadvantages attached to it. This is because baby chicks require so much care and attention as against older chickens. But, if this is done correctly, you are sure of reaping the rewards of taking proper care of them.

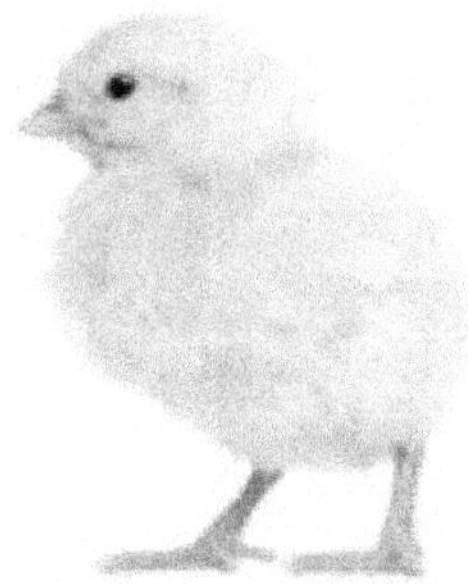

Bringing home

There are always several options that are made available to a poultry farmer. A poultry farmer can make choices as regards how to take care of his chickens. While it is always an exciting journey to bring new chicks from the incubator or purchase them from a local farm, they require so much care and attention.

If you desire to bring your chick home, it is advantageous to you as a farmer because you can decide to keep them just anywhere that pleases you. Nonetheless, it is essential to emphasize that these chicks will grow at a very rapid rate. Therefore, it is vital to make adequate space for them whilst they grow. As a matter of fact, between the period of four weeks, these chicks can also be taken outside to the chicken coop.

While chicks are still tender, it is necessary to protect their lives from keeping them far away from predators' reach and harsh weather conditions like a cold. A good way of keeping your chicks warm is to get a chick brooder. This would ensure that they are not affected by cold at such a tender stage of their development. Inasmuch as these chicks need to be kept warm and dry at all times, they also require ventilation. Some good ideas for keeping them dry whilst making proper ventilation available to them are the use of cardboard with holes on it or the use of a plastic storage bin. Whatever choice you settle for, it is proper to make adequate space for the chicks to roam around and explore their new environment.

As a budding poultry farmer, there are a number of things you may not know about chicks and their behavior. One of such things is the fact that baby chicks poop a lot. At that growing stage, all they do most of the time is feed and poop. This can be a lot of work for you as you are expected to keep the place clean and dry at all times as a damp environment would not be favorable to them. So, it is right to get appropriate absorbent bedding for them. This reduces the stress you would encounter in cleaning up the environment all the time. Some poultry farmers would instead settle for a newspaper as absorbent bedding. But, this would not do an excellent job in helping the chick environment stay dry. More so, it is wrong to use cedarwood shavings for the beddings of the chicks. This cedar wood shaving contains certain quantities of oil that is most likely going to affect the respiratory tract of the chicks at an older stage.

Baby chicks are naturally curious, and as such, they would desire to leap and fly whenever they have the opportunity to do so. As a poultry farmer, you need to understand that their behavior is prompted by curiosity and a willingness to explore their surroundings. So, it is expected that your chicks' environment is protected with a netting structure as this would keep them safe from escaping. In addition, your baby chicks are still growing, and this means they tend to eat so much food. So, you must make ample food and water available to them at all times. While there are quite a several foods you can feed your chicks, certain feeds are ideal for the growth of your baby chicks. If you want them to grow well and stay free from any form of disease, it is necessary to get the right type of food for their growth. Their drinking water is also very vital, but you would need to take special care in this regard.

Baby chicks are susceptible to various forms of injuries or situations that may most likely cost them their lives. To prevent this, get suitable drinking tubs that would make it difficult for your chicks to drown in them. The right type of drinking tub to get for your baby chicks is a chicken drinker. The chicken drinker helps ensure that your baby chicks in their large numbers will conveniently drink water without drowning in it. However, it is simply not enough to provide your baby chicks with water. You must pay attention to the content of their water. These chicks are very messy and can mess up their drinking water in no time. So, you can do them a lot of good by changing their water at regular intervals, ensuring that they drink clean water.

As a poultry farmer, you can help them experience less difficulty in feeding by providing them with shell grit. These shell grits are majorly found in pet stores and are very easy for your chicks to digest without passing through so much difficulty. This shell grit can be sprinkled on their food directly.

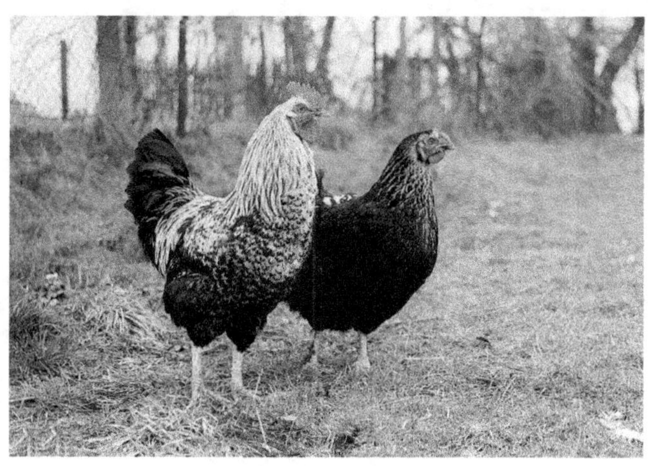

Quality and healthy chicks

The way you treat your chicks determines if they turn out healthy or not. You chicks can only be healthy when they are exposed to a suitable temperature. At their tender age, they rely on a convenient heat source to survive. This is why when a mother hen moves around with her little chicks, she always tucks them her plumage. The reason is that they need to heat source to keep them warm at all times. This stage would continue until they are older and require less heat. Maintaining a good heat source for your chicks requires the use of an infrared heat lamp. The heat should be placed above the heads of your chicks to give them much-desired warmth. Even in the choice of an infrared heat lamp, it is proper to get one that enables them to sleep properly rather than distract them from having adequate rest. Therefore, it is necessary to pay close attention to your chicks' health and behavior as it would enable you to take appropriate actions when necessary.

An example is if you notice your chicks are crowding behind a heat source. This indicates that they are cold and require warmth. If this happens, you can choose to lower the heat lamp or put in an additional heat source to give them warmth in the room. Also, if you notice that your chicks are always favoring the edge of their brooder, then chances are that they feel too hot and are trying to get away from the heat source as far as possible. If this is the case, it is essential that you conveniently find a way of creating a balance within their living area so that they don't become uncomfortable.

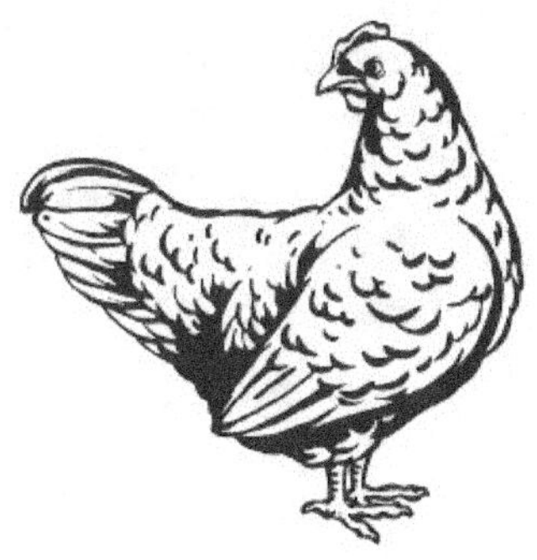

Healthy chickens thrive on good feed. If you want your chicks to be healthy and possess good quality, be sure to feed them with the right type of meal that is instrumental to their growth and development. The ideal feed to get for chicks is known as starter feeds. These feeds contain the necessary nutrients that the chicks desire to grow properly. Starter feeds can in two different forms, that is, crumbles and mash.

Before you feed your chicks with any type of feed, ensure that you go through the necessary guidelines and follow them to the letter. It would be stipulated the right time to feed your baby chicks and how long they should be fed.

Furthermore, some manufacturers produce starter feeds as a starter/grower combination. These combinations can be fed to your chicks for a longer time as against just the starter feed. Also, you can choose to give your chicks additional feeds so as to keep them healthy at all times. Without a doubt, the starter feed contains all that they require to grow properly, but you can also choose to feed them with worms and even kitchen scraps.

You may wonder just how much quantity of chicken feed becomes too small or too big for your chicks, right? There are no rules for feeding your baby chicks! You only need to make sure that they have food available to them at all times. This would keep them feeling healthy and active. Moreover, your chicks would like always eat whenever they feel hungry, and immediately they are satisfied, they would let the food be. So, with your chick, there is no such term as "overeating." As a matter of fact, it is always better to make food available to them rather than deprive them of food and make them malnourished.

Common diseases

Chicks are susceptible to various forms of diseases. Interestingly, with the appropriate cleanliness of their environment, these chicks can stay away from diseases. Some of the diseases are highly preventable, so it is vital that you recognize each disease's symptoms and know how to keep your flock safe.

Some examples of these diseases are:

Brooder pneumonia: A damp environment commonly brings about this disease. Symptoms of this disease include gasping for air, nasal discharge, head twisting, and inability to balance. The only way to keep them away from this disease is to keep the environment clean at all times. The treatment of this disease is also readily available and can be administered to sick chicks to make them feel better.

Coccidiosis: This disease is caused as a result of the wrong consumption of a certain thing. Chickens are fond of picking at anything they come across, including poop. This affects their intestines and causes them to fall ill. This disease causes their poo to change color to become either red or orange, and in some cases, it is accompanied by mucus in their poop. The resultant effect is that your chicks become withdrawn and less active. Your chick may not likely be affected by this disease, but they will certainly not be as productive or energetic as they should have been. To prevent Coccidiosis, it is necessary always to change your chicks' bedding and ensure that they are dry.

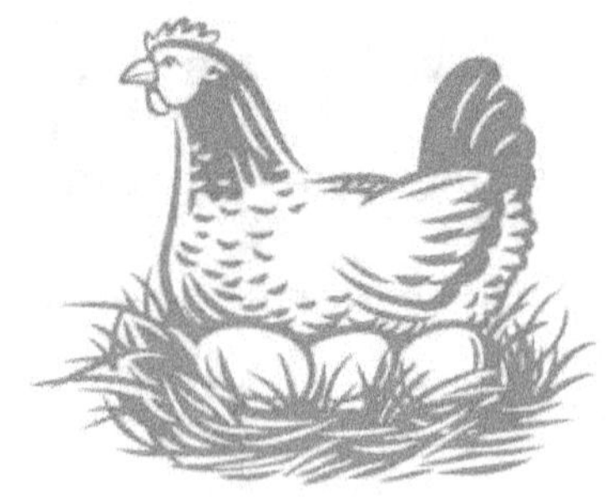

Infectious bronchitis: This is a common disease associated with chicken, commonly referred to as the "Chicken cold." The symptoms of this disease include coughing, difficulty in breathing, nasal discharge, and huddling together. This disease is hazardous because if a chick has a cold, it is most likely going to affect the other chicks. Unfortunately, below six weeks of age, chicks are most likely to be affected by this disease, which causes the highest number of deaths. There are numerous vaccines that are significant in preventing infectious bronchitis. Still, the best way of keeping your chicks safe from this disease is to provide them with an appropriate heat temperature. Moreover, when chicks are more likely to get cold, they become susceptible to other forms of diseases.

Omphalitis: This disease is caused by the navel of the chicken being affected just after hatching. It implies that some bacteria may have just being pushed into the eggshell after hatching. Some common symptoms are swollen navel and a distended stomach. This is commonly caused by poor sanitation of the incubator or the hatching environment. the best way to prevent this disease is to favor a clean environment and clean the navel of the chicks with a quantity of iodine.

Salmonella: This disease leads to the death of chicks. Some of the symptoms are diarrhea, fatigue, and loss of appetite. While this disease can also be dangerous to humans, it is carried out by chickens. An affected chick can be treated with the aid of an antibiotic. To play safe and prevent this disease's presence amongst your flock, ensure you purchase your flocks from good and tested hatcheries.

Rotgut: Chicks that are affected by this disease always have offensive-smelling diarrhea and listlessness. It is usually contracted through overcrowding. So, whenever you overcrowd your chicks, you put them at risk of contracting rotgut. This disease can be prevented by administering antibiotics in their drinking water.

The good news is that these diseases can be prevented or controlled when the chicken coop is kept clean. In addition to this, before introducing a chick to the chicken coop, make sure that it is adequately isolated from the others.

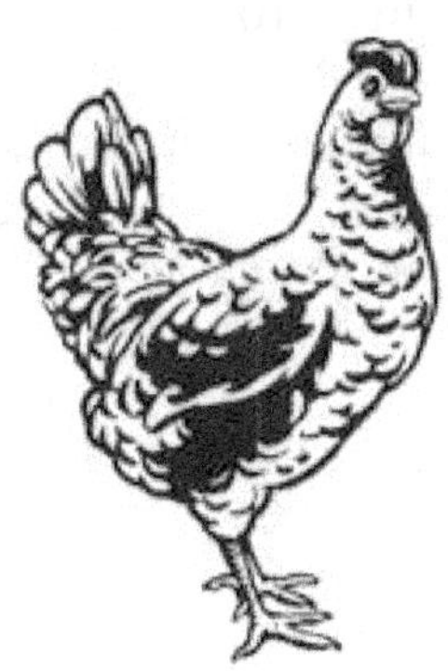

Deworming chicks

When chicks have too many worms in their bodies, it would not only affect their health and abilities to produce eggs, in worse case scenarios, it could also lead to death. An important question to ask is, "How do I know my chicks need deworming?" The environment where the chicks are kept can give you the insight to know if your chicks need deworming or not. If the chicken area is always covered in poop, be rest assured that your chicks will feed on this poop. Sadly, some of these poops contain worm eggs. So, when the chicks eat them, they are confident of consuming these worms into their bodies. Some common worms that affect chicks are roundworms and flatworms. These worms can be controlled by deworming your chickens.

Although some poultry farmers rely on the use of natural items such as garlic, cucumber, and squash to prevent these worms' growth, this has proved more effective than administering the medication on them. However, it is believed that deworming chicks would eventually make them resistant to the medication. So, the best deal is to avoid any circumstance that would make the chicks vulnerable and be affected by worms. These include cleaning the coop regularly, keeping their feeders and drinking tubs as well.

CHAPTER FIVE
FEED, WATER, AND TREATS

Chickens require special feed that is highly concentrated in the nutrients that their bodies need for growth. With this, it becomes easy to achieve the right type of egg and meat production desired.

Balanced nutrition for chickens

What does balanced nutrition for chicken mean?

The nutritional needs of chickens vary at different phases of their growth. As such, when chicks are newly born, they require feeds that contain good portions of proteins. These proteins are instrumental in their development and growth. For chickens about 8-18 weeks, their nutritional needs require less protein as against the newly born chicks.

When chickens reach the stage where they produce eggs, their nutritional needs differ significantly. There are a lot more requirements on what their bodies need to grow properly. As such, their feeds would involve layer rotation as soon as they begin to lay eggs. Also, their feeds need to contain more calcium and a good quantity of grit as well. It is common knowledge that as soon as chickens begin to age, their ability to produce eggs dramatically diminishes. The only way to ensure that they produce eggs for you is to start feeding them with the appropriate feeds at a very early age. This would help them stay active and productive for you.

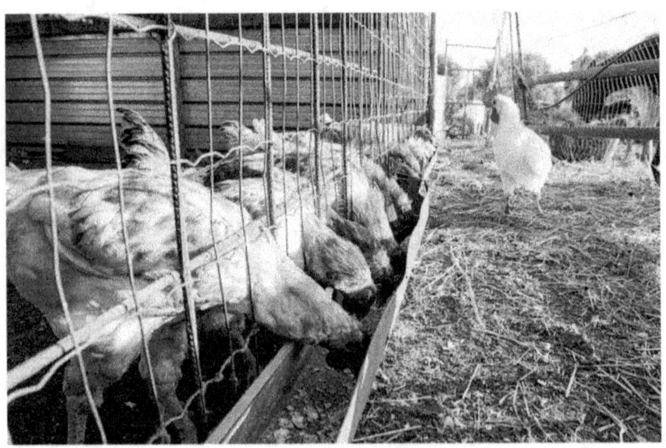

As soon as your chickens start producing eggs, it is important to feed them with layers feed. Layers feed differs from broilers' feed. The difference in the two eggs is as a result of the uses of those eggs. When eggs are solely meant for human consumption, the chickens are fed with layers eggs. But, if the eggs are for the purpose of hatching, the chickens are fed with broiler feeds. Also, it is possible to give them a supplementary treat by adding ground oyster shells to their feed. As a poultry farmer, you need to monitor the quality of the eggshells that your chicks produce. With this, you would know if they require ground oyster shells in their feed or not. In cases where the chickens produce eggs with cracked shells, it is best to feed them with an additional ground oyster shell.

Therefore, chickens that produce eggs need to eat feeds that contain a higher quantity of protein.

There are supplementary treats that can be offered to chickens to increase their production of eggs. These meals are:

- Greens and vegetables
- Mealworms
- Fruits and watermelon
- Sunflower seeds and so on

These treats are a great way to improve the egg production of your chickens. They boost egg production and make their eggs more nutritious. It is normal to feed your chickens with layer feeds. But, there is also a need to supplement their feed with something extra. The fact remains that chickens that are adequately fed will always produce a good amount of eggs than chickens that are not.

Toxic plants and food

Chickens are always eager to find out things for themselves. Often, they are always seen scratching the ground in their quest to find something for them to eat. Irrespective of the fact that they are fed well, they still desire to fend for themselves by getting something they can eat independently. The negative effect of this is that these chickens are exposed to harmful plants that may affect their overall health. Some of the plants that are considered toxic to chickens are:

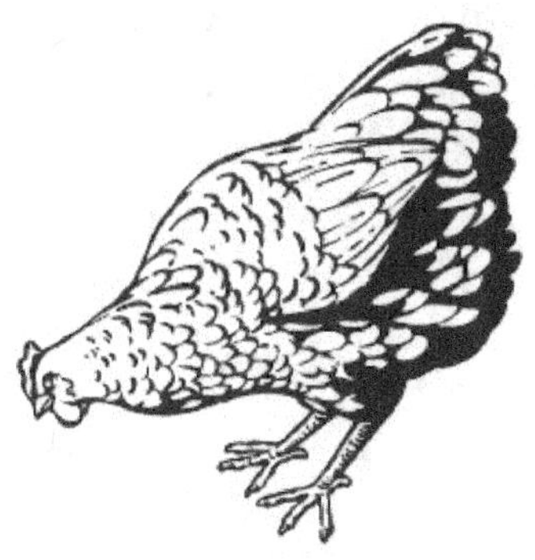

Solanaceae: These are plants that belong to the nightshade family. They contain a certain compound which is referred to as solanine. Examples of plants in this category are potatoes, tomatoes, and so on. These plants are considered toxic to chickens. The only type when the compound contained in these foods is reduced is when they are cooked. If these foods are cooked, it is okay to feed your chickens, but if not, they are very harmful to your chicken's health.

Onions: These are also toxic plants to chickens, especially when given to them in large quantities. These plants can cause anemia, jaundice and can also affect the red blood cells of the chickens.

Avocado pears: These plants are beneficial to humans but can adversely affect the health of chickens. It contains a substance known as persin. This toxic can affect the health of the chicken and cause their heart to stop functioning properly.

Apple's seeds: Apple is a great plant, but the seeds can become toxic to chickens. These plants contain a substance known as cyanide. This substance can affect your chickens. It is advised to feed your chickens with any part of the apple apart from the seed.

Citrus: If these plants are given to chickens in moderation, they would cause no harm. But, when they are fed to chickens, they bring about a reduction in their egg production.

Raw beans: Your chickens should not be fed with dry beans. These dry beans contain a substance that is toxic to your chickens. If you must feed your chicken with beans, it needs to be cooked beans and not raw.

Sugar: Sugar is not considered appropriate for humans. When humans consume too much quantity of sugar, it will affect their health. This is also applicable to chickens. When these chickens are fed with sugar, it would affect their ability to produce eggs properly because they may properly become overweight.

Excessive salts: When there is too much salt contained in chicken feeds, it would most likely affect their bodies. Chickens are not good at consuming salt, and excessive salt in their feed can cause salt poisoning and make them less healthy than they ought to be. Naturally, chickens do not favor salt, and any attempt to do this will affect them immensely.

Moldy food: It is important to stay as far away from moldy foods as possible. These foods are toxic to your chickens and should be avoided at all costs. Sadly, this moldy food can affect your chickens so much so that they may even die as a result of it. Feeding your chicken will overripe fruits, wilted vegetables and stale bread is not a problem. The only time it becomes a problem is when these foods contain molds.

There are also a handful of garden plants that are considered toxic to your chickens. Though your chickens may not enjoy these plants as a result of their smell, it is also best to keep them as far away from these toxic plants as far as possible. Some examples of these toxic garden plants are:

- Fern
- Ground ivy
- Horseradish
- Ivy
- Lily of the valley
- Bloodroot
- Castor bean
- Hemlock

Medical care of chickens

The health of your chicken is very important and should not be taken for granted. The well-being of your chicken depends on how you care for them. When you pay close attention to your chicken, it becomes easy for you to detect if something is wrong with them or not. Peradventure something is wrong with them, you can easily find out the best way to treat them before they affect others or die due to the illness. Also, if any of your chicken is ill or experiencing a certain type of illness, it is advisable to isolate them for a while until they are fully recovered. Even in isolating your sick chicken, you need to make sure that you provide them with adequate food and water to keep them going and speed up the recovery process.

Ensure you contact your medical professional to assist you in giving help to your chickens. Your chickens require a veterinary doctor's assistance to access them and give them an appropriate medication that would help them feel better. As a matter of fact, it is even preferable to contact your veterinary doctor before even setting up your chicken coop.

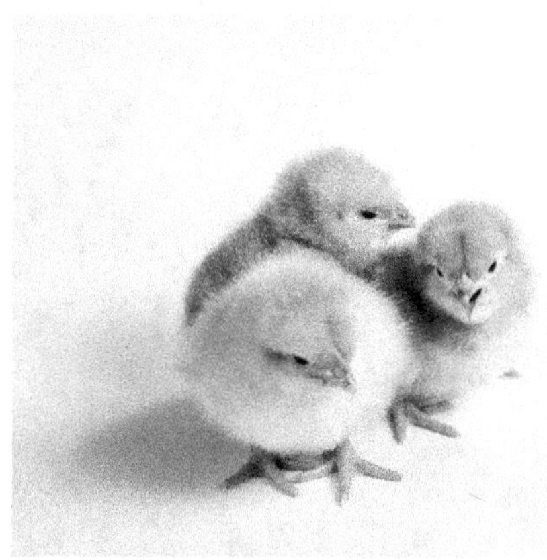

Symptoms your chickens are ill

You would notice certain symptoms in your chickens that would indicate that they are not feeling well. Immediately you discover any of these symptoms, and you should speak with a Vet to proffer the right type of solution to your chickens' medical condition. Some of the symptoms may include:

- Lice and mite
- Loss of feather
- Respiratory issues
- A change in their stool
- Loss of energy
- Poor movement
- Poor appetite
- Stunted growth

While it is almost difficult to control an outbreak of disease amongst your chickens, it is necessary to do what is right to prevent the outbreak of the disease among your chickens. This is because it is easier to prevent the disease among your chickens than to control it. If you keep your chicken environment clean and provide clean water for them, there are good chances you are keeping your chickens safe from any disease outbreak. Unfortunately, even with all of the regular checks on these chickens, they still seem to fall ill and become susceptible to various diseases. But, the importance of a routine inspection of your flock is to identify any illness or disease and take immediate action to control the spread of the diseases. Suppose, as a poultry farmer, you fail to pay medical attention to your chickens, and they become affected by various types of diseases. In that case, you may lose them as the authorities may require that you terminate all of them to prevent a further outbreak of such disease.

CHAPTER SIX
PROS AND CONS OF RAISING CHICKENS

Every conscious business individual needs to understand the advantages and disadvantages that are associated with a chosen business venture. It is the knowledge of the gains and losses involved in the business that helps poultry farmers devise suitable and reliable means of handling their flocks. Yet, the pros should outweigh the cons of the business; else, it may leave you with unpleasant memories.

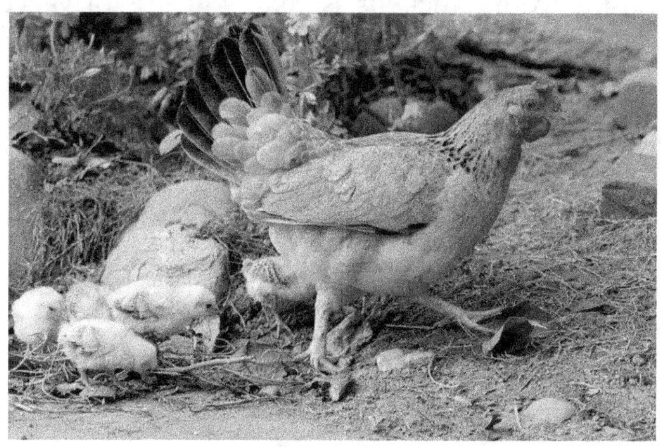

Pros of raising chickens

The production of more nutritious eggs: Without a doubt, eggs produced from your poultry farm will also taste better than those purchased from local stores. If the emphasis is on the consumption of nutritious eggs, then it would do you a lot of good to consume eggs produced by chickens you have raised. The differences in the taste of the chickens' eggs are brought about by quite a number of reasons ranging from the type of feed they are fed with, the kind of space made available to them, and your intent to raise the chickens. An advantage of being a poultry farmer and raising your chickens is that you are privileged to monitor what they consume and feed them properly. Now, when you purchase eggs from stores, you have no idea about the type of feed and space the chicken that produced the egg was exposed to. So, how can you ascertain the quality of the egg to be consumed?

You can profit off it: AS a poultry farmer, raising your chickens can be a good way for you to make some extra money. When your chickens produce eggs, you can choose to sell off the eggs and earn some money from them. For example, if you have about 20 hens, there are higher chances that about 14 hens would lay eggs in a day. When you sell off your eggs, you are sure of making extra income to take care of your needs. Fortunately, there are lots of individuals that are willing to pay to consume quality eggs. Since you train chickens, this is an excellent opportunity for you to make some money.

Varieties of egg color: As a poultry farmer, you may have different breeds of chicken in your chicken loop. This gives you the advantage of having different colors of eggs on your farm. The various colors of eggs can range from brown, white, and in some cases, blue and green.

Raising chickens is a good way to relieve stress: While there are common pets and animals, it is no news that some pets are friendly than others. Chickens are one of such friendly pets. If you are desirous of letting go of the stress you feel, your chickens can produce the much-needed relief you seek. Naturally, chickens are a curious lot. They would always hop around in your presence and may even come running towards you if they think you want to give them something to eat.

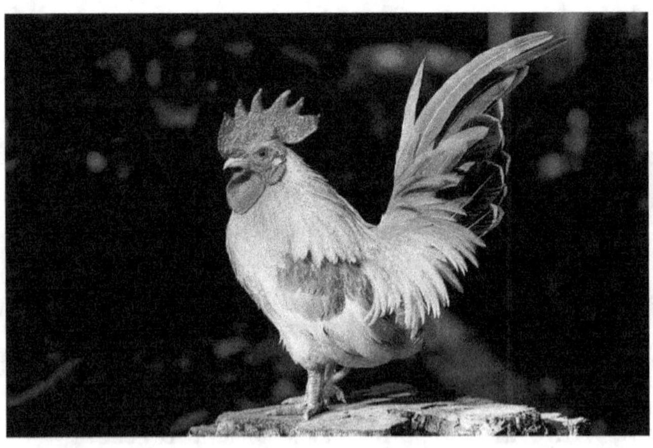

The production of meat: Of course, chickens are good sources of protein and healthy fat. Chickens are advantageous in that they are essential in the production of tasty meat. The best way to ensure that you utilize the production of meat from chickens is to avoid any form of emotional connection with them. This is because when you are emotionally connected to these chickens, it becomes difficult for you to kill them. Aside from personal consumption, you can also decide to sell off the meat produced from chicken to individuals interested in its consumption.

It is a good source of fertilizer: The droppings from chickens are good sources of fertilizer. This dropping can either be added to your garden to make it blossom and stay healthy, or it could be sold away to other farmers that require its use.

Cons of raising chickens

Its maintenance can be pretty expensive: Seeing the number of advantages associated with raising chickens, it is also expected that some disadvantages are attached to its use. Generally, chickens are known to be messy as they always create a mess of their environment. Thus, as a poultry farmer, you are saddled with the responsibility of changing the materials used in the construction of their chicken coop and cleaning up the place regularly. If this is not done, they would be exposed to various forms of illness and predators. To clean your chicken coop, it is encouraged that you favor the use of sanitary materials and also protect yourself in the process.

It is a demanding process: Poultry farmers are always expected to look it for the chickens. Sometimes, this may even interfere with personal choices or activities. For example, you are expected to make sure that your chickens are well-rested at night to keep them away from harm's way.

It is your responsibility to ensure that they have enough food, water, and grit at their disposal in the same vein. For your chickens to grow healthy and stay happy, adequate provision of all of these would make it possible. Failure to do this would only mean that you would not make your desired profit off them. While this is a necessity for their growth, they can also infringe upon your movement and choices. Thus, making you feel less satisfied and pleased.

Finance: Raising chickens is also very financially demanding. As a poultry farmer, you would spend a reasonable amount of money to ensure your chickens' comfort. This includes purchasing feeds for them from when they were hatched until the period they die. Besides, you would also require money for their medication and to take care of other chicken-related needs. The financial involvement of this activity may take a negative toll on your finances if you are not financially capable.

Fortunately, the pros of raising chickens outweigh its cons. As such, this is a good and exciting business activity.

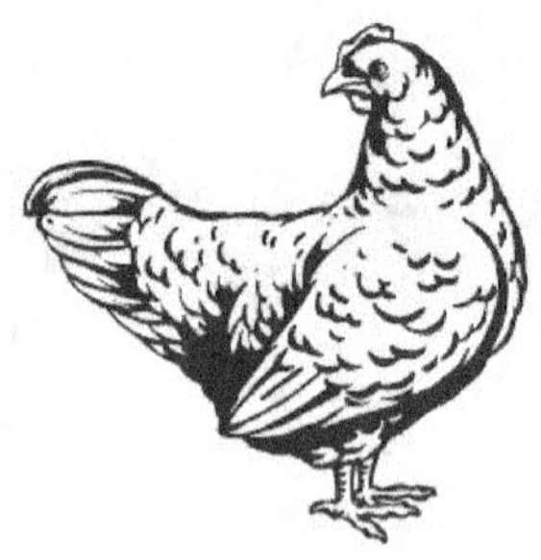

Hen routine management

Hens are known to be the female chickens that are significant in the production of eggs. It is also believed that they are sexually ready to aid the production of eggs. From the age of 20 weeks, these hens are expected to start laying eggs. The act of laying eggs is always regular until the egg production reduces when they get to about 75 weeks.

Hen management involves being knowledgeable about what they require to stay active and productive during their laying period. Thus, their caging system feeds, and medication should not be taken for granted at that stage. The caging system that is used for hens in recent times is the California system. This cage system is better than the traditional caging system because it does not require so much space as compared to the traditional caging system. Also, it protects the hens from contracting various forms of diseases from one another.

The ability of hens to produce eggs depends on how they are taken care of. This means that poultry farmers are expected to provide good electricity sources for their chickens and also make sure that they do not lack the necessary feeds that are a prerequisite for their egg production. It is also crucial that in a suitable place to keep these hens, the land space must be elevated to prevent any situation where their environment is flooded with water or a place prone to predators. The amount of feed to be given to hens is very important. It is suggested that the hens should be fed for minimum of two times a day.

When all of these conditions are religiously met, there are good chances that the hens will not only be healthy but would also produce nutritious eggs as well.

Coop clean up

For the health of your chickens, it is important to keep their coop clean at all times. Most importantly, you should also keep yourself clean while doing that! What are the various ways of keeping the chicken coop clean? They are:

Take out the beddings: Your chickens would always leave their beddings in a mess. They are not humans and would not be irritated by it. But, you are right? Well, you can make their environment clean by taking it upon yourself to look out for them at all times! How? With the aid of hand gloves and perhaps a face mask, take out everything in their coops, such as their drinking tubs and feeders. When you have carefully removed all of these, take out their beddings. Now that you have taken their beddings outside, get a paint scraper and scrape off any unpleasant substance on the beddings.

Take off the debris: This is the second step of the cleaning process. At this stage, it is expected that you take out the debris in the chicken coop by scraping off the debris. If you encounter any challenging or complicated debris, make use of your coop cleaner and scrub thoroughly until you have successfully taken it off.

Thoroughly rinse and repeat the process: After scrubbing the coop, you would have to rinse it off with the aid of water. This would help to take off whatever dirt that is still left in the coop. This can be done with the aid of boiling water and some quantity of apple cider vinegar. Ensure you also clean out the feeders and drinking tubs with the use of apple cider vinegar.

Get fresh bedding. At this stage, the chicken coop must have been dried thoroughly. Now, get fresh bedding for your chickens. Perhaps, the old bedding is no longer attractive and already an eyesore. A change of bedding would leave your chickens feeling healthy and happy.

Replace the items: You must have taken out the feeders and drinking tub outside. As soon as your chicken coop is looking all neat and attractive, it is time for you to replace every item that you had taken out in the cleaning process. If there is any damaged item you can do without, it is necessary to avoid using it again.

Most importantly, never joke with your health, even in the cleaning process. As such, after cleaning out your chicken coop, ensure you wash your hands thoroughly to prevent any spread.

Seasonal considerations

On a seasonal basis, your chickens require special consideration. This also involves that you get involved in doing certain tasks for them. This would help their transition during various climatic conditions.

Winter season: This is characterized by rain and snowfall. While this is not too much for humans to handle, it can affect the overall health of your chickens. During this period, your chickens are prone to be frostbitten. This can be adequately taken care of by applying a small quantity of Vaseline to their combs. Another issue that may likely experience is freezing. To prevent them from freezing and saving their lives, ensure that they do not provide water to them during the night. It is also important to keep their resting places very warm. There is no better soothing feeling than the thought of coming back to a warm resting place during the winter season.

Spring season: This is usually a more preferred season considering the fact that the gardens would be looking colorful and attractive and interesting; your hens may be ready to lay eggs. While this is a comforting thought, it is still necessary to look after your chickens' health. This season is an appropriate time for you to clean out your chicken coop thoroughly. This would give you the privilege of making your desired changes in the coop. It is no surprise that at this time, your hens may show symptoms of broodiness. The best way to handle this situation is to ensure that you collect their eggs appropriately and discourage this habit amongst them.

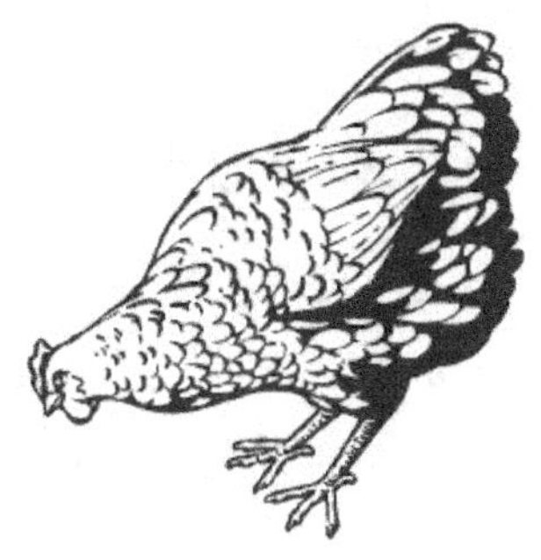

Summer season: This period may negatively affect your chickens, which is why it is essential that you consider some basic tips. Your chickens will probably be stressed and uncomfortable during the summer season as a result of the heat temperature. A good way of keeping them cool and active is by providing shade for them to rest and also make provision of an adequate source of water. More so, you can feed them with lots of frozen fruits and vegetables. They would sure love the feel of something frozen in the heat temperature! If you notice that the weather is exceedingly hot, get a bowl and fill it with some quantity of water. Some of your chickens would quickly stand on the water as a means of reducing their body heat. It is at this season that lice and mice are prevalent. You can control the effect of these parasites by preventing their presence.

Autumn season: This is a period where your chickens are most likely going to feel relaxed. Yet, you need to ensure that they stay healthy throughout the season. How? Molts are very common during the autumn season. You can stop it from affecting your chickens by giving them a good quantity of their dietary needs and leaving them healthy.

Common chicken problems

Chickens also experience one form of a health problem or another. These chicken problems can be kept at bay by feeding them with the much-needed nutrients and supplements essential for their growth. Even while making provision for their nutrients and supplements, it is also a wise thought to administer antibiotics on them as this can be an excellent way to prevent cholera, coccidiosis, fowl pox, avian influenza, Newcastle disease, and salmonella. If, as a poultry farmer, you take into consideration their health problems and stay abreast of any health challenges they encounter, you would indeed witness minimal or no losses whatsoever.

Cannibalism

In poultry, cannibalism is also known as aggressive pecking. Chickens are commonly known to peck at the ground, especially as they are eager to feed or discover whatever it is that arouses their curiosity. Since this is a natural tendency, why does it seem to be an issue amongst chickens? Well, cannibalism is destructive because it is mainly used by older chickens to intimidate the young ones and is even worse when any form of injury occurs.

Cannibalism is usually characterized by plucking the feathers of other chickens. This may become worse when the affected chickens are unable to defend themselves. Research has proven that various variables may be a cause for such attitudes amongst chickens. These variables range from poor ventilation, nutrient deficiency, hot temperature, amongst others. If cannibalism amongst chickens is not kept minimal, it can become a learned behavior and eventually a habit promoted amongst all the chickens.

A good way of preventing cannibalism amongst your chickens is to make use of good husbandry practices. It is also suggested that their environment's lighting should be made so that they would be comfortable in their coop. Trimming the beak of these chickens is also a good way of controlling cannibalism in your chickens. This behavior amongst your chickens can also be controlled if you are quick to remove sick or injured chickens. Another way is to feed them with abundant fiber. When their feeds are packed with fiber, they will become less cannibalistic.

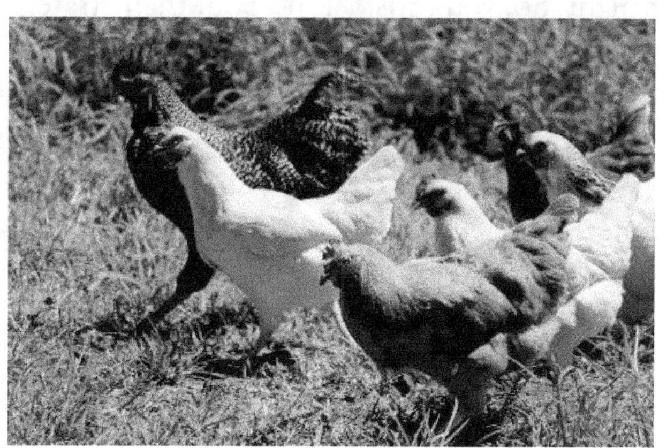

How to protect your chickens from predators

If you don't protect your chickens from predators, who will? Of course, your chickens may also devise ways of protecting themselves from predators, but no one would do it better than you!

The right way to guarantee the safety of your chickens is to identify their predators. Except you discover the threats to your chickens, you may never be able to keep them away from harm. These predators can attack at any time of the day or night. So, you must learn about their strategies and devise appropriate means of handling the situation.

After identifying your predators, it is necessary to prevent your chicken from their grasp. This you can do by building a good fence that would keep them safe since they protect your chicken from being a nuisance to your neighbors. Another means of protecting your chickens from predators is to make use of mesh in constructing their environment. Ensure you leave the mesh with tiny holes such that predators would find it difficult to get through. It would also do you a whole lot of good to train your chickens on how to retire for the night. When you instill this habit in them, they will find it easy to always retire to their coop in the evening, and this is a safe way of keeping them safe from predator's attack.

As a poultry farmer, it is pertinent that you get a good site for your chicken coop. This involves making a clear survey of the environment and making sure it is free from any harm or imposing danger. When this is done, your chickens would worry less about encountering predatory attacks. You can also indirectly invite predators to attack your chickens by feeding them unknowingly. So, to avert such situations, only feed your chickens with adequate meals for their feeding and feed them accordingly.

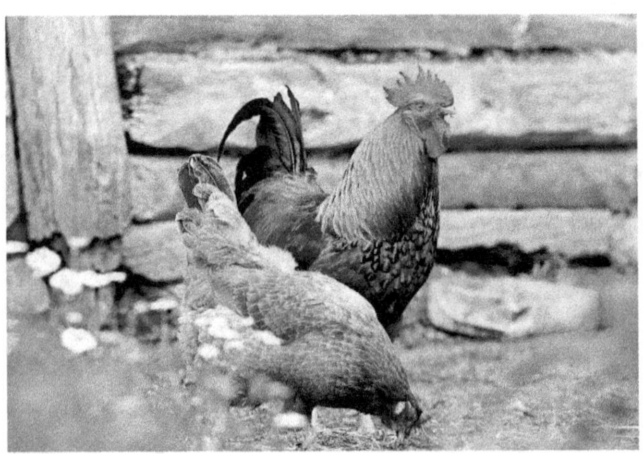

CHAPTER SEVEN
GATHERING EGGS

A commonly asked question is, "How often do I gather eggs laid by my chickens?" it has been clearly stated in the earlier course of this book that chickens lay one egg in a day. However, it is also essential to note that chickens lay their eggs at different times of the day. While a chicken may lay her egg in the morning, another chicken can lay eggs in the evening. As a poultry farmer, you are saddled with the responsibility of performing a routine check on their coop so that you can pick up any egg that is laid. Whatever reason you are gathering eggs for, you must gather the eggs regularly and keep them in a safe place. An advantage of gathering eggs regularly is that it saves you the loss of having a cracked or damaged egg. It also helps you gather more clean, fresh eggs from your chicken coop.

Nesting boxes

Nesting boxes are a safe and secure place where your chickens can lay their eggs. Just as every mother is protective of her offspring, hens also act in the same way. This is where it is often a surprise how chickens identify places to lay their eggs. Sometimes, their choices remain a mystery to poultry farmers as they try to make out the reason behind their choices. But, chickens are assured of having a safe place where they can lay their eggs with nesting boxes. Fortunately, nesting boxes are not a mystery or something difficult to make as they can be made from just anything. But, for their comfort, it is crucial to give them something where they can perch for a while before sitting on their eggs. To make them more comfortable, it is necessary to put some sand or straw in their nesting boxes. The number of nesting boxes you require in your poultry farm depends on the number of chickens you have.

Thus, a nesting box is considered sufficient for about three to four chickens, and this makes provision for space for the birds. These nesting boxes' sizes vary, but the least size should be about 5 inches. The only time chickens require a nesting box is when they are about sixteen to seventeen weeks. No, you may wonder how best to construct your nesting boxes for the chickens. While your nesting boxes do not necessarily need to have a cover, if it does, it is a good way of making your hens feel safe and comfortable. Nesting boxes can be designed with the presence of a divider and can also work better without any. Protecting the eggs laid by these chickens also implies that you secure the nesting boxes where these eggs are laid. Sometimes, the chickens may need to flap their wings or move around. If the nesting boxes are not secure, they may cause the nesting boxes to flip, and then the eggs will break. To protect your eggs and the hen, it is vital to have the nesting box securely placed.

Another factor to be considered is the type of material used in the construction of the nesting box. The suitable materials that are not susceptible to bacteria are plastic and metal material. Although it is ubiquitous to see wooden nesting boxes, this material is not the best. These nesting boxes should not be too placed high above the grounds. Instead, it should be placed in a position that makes the chicken comfortable. It is important to place these nesting boxes very close to the window for ventilation in the same vein. In cases where it becomes difficult or expensive to afford nesting boxes, it is suggested that poultry owners improvise by making use of buckets. As a rule, your nesting boxes should be kept within the confines of your chicken loop. This would help you encounter less difficulty in monitoring the chickens and how they lay their eggs

Well, it is not a surprise of chickens decide to sleep in their nesting boxes. But, this should be avoided before it becomes a norm for them.

Nesting boxes should also be kept clean and away from dirt. These boxes also need to be made accessible to you so that it can make it easier for you to collect eggs regularly.

Reasons your chickens stopped laying eggs

Are you bordered your chickens have stopped laying eggs? Do you hope to find out the reasons to make the right corrections? Well, this is the time when the various factors that are responsible for the inability of your chickens to lay eggs are discussed!

Some of the reasons are:

A change in their diet: Rather than concern yourself with unnecessary worry about why your chickens stopped laying eggs, pay attention to their diet. Did you make any changes to their diet? If you did, this might be the cause of their inability to lay eggs again. A change in your chickens' diet may cause them to stop laying eggs or could even bring about a reduction in the number of eggs they produce in a day. If this is your story, then go back to feeding them the right feed!

Insufficient light: If the lighting system in the chicken coop is poor, do not expect your chickens to lay eggs like they used to. Chickens need the presence of an adequate amount of daylight for them to produce eggs. Also, different seasons can bring about a change in their abilities to produce eggs. So, if you notice that they produce eggs well in a particular season as against another, it has nothing to do with you. When the season is right, they will produce more eggs.

Broody hens: Even if you feed your chickens with a good diet and expose her to natural light, she would find it difficult to lay eggs if she is a broody hen. Broody hens are always desirous of hatching their eggs. This is why they sit on their eggs and try to hatch after 21 days. Well, if this is what your hen does, be rest assured that she will refuse to lay eggs, and this does you no good. So, to avert this, ensure you discourage this habit by picking eggs regularly.

Additions: When you make any slight change in their location or introduce a new chicken in their midst, this can cause their egg production to reduce drastically. Not to worry, after your chickens have accepted the new flock in their midst, they would go back to laying eggs just like they used to.

The type of chicken breed: While people seem to believe that hens possessed an innate ability to lay eggs, it is important to emphasize that certain chicken breeds will lay eggs slower than others. Thus, it is erroneous to complain when your chickens are not laying eggs. The first thing you should identify is their laying patterns and understanding why it works that way.

Age: Age affects the production of eggs. As such, the older a hen gets, the more difficult it is to lay eggs. When hens newly begin to lay eggs, they always produce reasonable quantities of eggs. But, as soon as they start to age, their production diminishes, and this may begin to get you worried. Well, if your hen is probably aged, this may be a factor that has prompted her inability to lay eggs for you.

The presence of disease: There is no way you can compare the activities and strength of a healthy chicken to one which is not. Thus, when your chicken is healthy, they will most likely produce a good number of eggs than when they are not. Various factors such as cold, parasites, and molds can affect your chickens and bring about a reduction in their egg production.

If your chicken experiences any of the aforementioned, then that explains the sudden reduction in their egg production and even the cause of their inability to lay eggs properly.

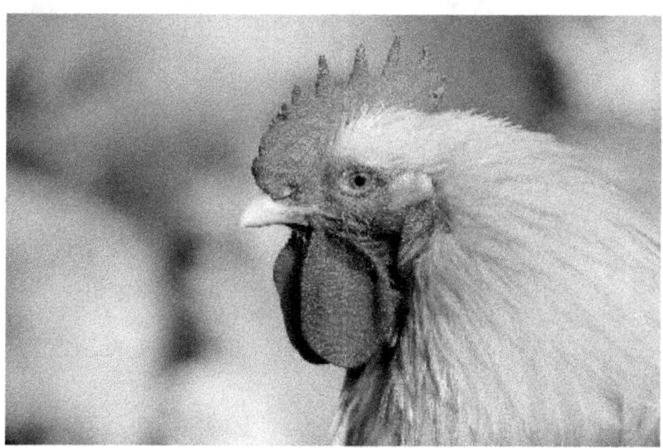

CHAPTER EIGHT
GETTING TO KNOW YOUR HENS

As a poultry farmer, you are probably enjoying the company of your chickens. It is incredible to watch these creatures roam about your garden and use their beak to till the ground in their quest to find something to eat. Well, you would be unable to achieve all that you need when you have successfully mastered how your chickens behave. Although your chickens may take a longer time to get used to you with time, they definitely would. To make this a reality, it is important that you play your role in making this possible. This is also possible when you make out time to learn more about your chickens and how they behave.

Behavior and psychology of chickens

Psychology of chickens means having the right knowledge or understanding of how your chickens behave or act under certain conditions. Except you exert conscious effort to understand the psychology behind these chickens' attitudes, you may find it difficult to treat them the right way. Some of the things you probably had no ideas concerning your chickens are:

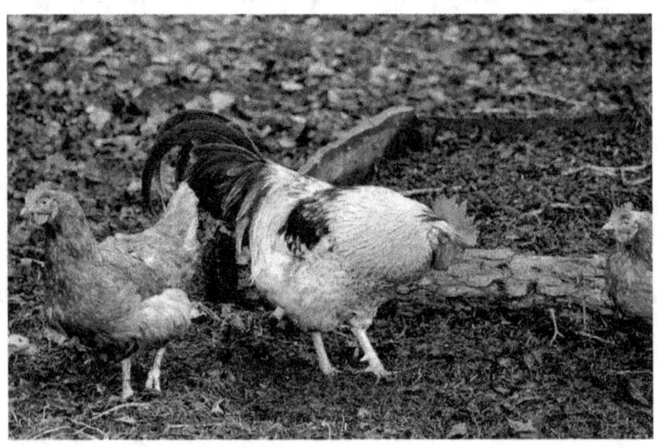

They teach one another: Is it not fascinating to watch a mother hen lead her children wherever she goes? Have you noticed how defensive she acts when you get too close to her chicks? This is the same character humans exhibit when they feel the society wants to come in between them and their children. The mother hen does not just carry her children along with her wherever she goes; she also teaches them in the process. This is why whenever she is using her beak to till the ground, her children watch her, and with time they begin to imitate her. Even after she does, she allows them to eat up whatever it is she had found while digging at the ground. Doing this, she teaches them to fend for themselves. Amazing, isn't it?

They recognize their owners: This may come as a surprise to you, especially as you wonder if they won't forget you in the twinkle of an eye. Well, chickens are not forgetful. This is why you must train them as soon as possible. By training them, you make it difficult for them to forget about you. You must have noticed that whenever you step into their coop to feed them or give them water, they start making noises. Sometimes, they even rally around you without any form of fear. Well, the reason behind such behavior is because they know you own them.

The combs of hens are usually big when they are about to lay eggs: Well, you may not have noticed this before now. But, their combs get bigger when they are about to lay their eggs. As a matter of fact, there are other signs that a hen shows just before she lays eggs. Their comb getting larger is just one of those signs. Another sign she shows is that she becomes very submissive.

Hens communicate to their young ones before they hatch them: Are you surprises? You probably didn't expect this. But, this is true! When the chicks are still in the eggs, the mother hen can communicate to them through talking and clucking. As time goes on, these chicks understand what their mom does and start to respond. This is why it is prevalent to see that chicks share a special bond with their moms. Interestingly, when these chicks hatch, they experience no difficulty recognizing their mom's voice even when she is not close back. This behavior is a result of the communication that had already taken place when they were yet hatched.

Chickens possess speed: A good majority of the chicken breeds are swift. Sometimes, you may attempt to catch them, and before you know it, they have entirely left your presence to another location. This ability they possess keeps them away from predators and helps them always stay safe from any form of danger.

They enjoy playing a lot: You must have noticed that your chickens jump around a lot. Well, they enjoy playing, and this is why they appear restless. For a majority of the time, chickens are running around, scraping the ground, or jostling one another. Their playfulness triggers such an attitude amongst them.

Chickens follow a hierarchical order: Humans are not the only beings that obey hierarchical order; even chickens do as well. This is why you must have seen two cocks jousting each other. This is done to indicate territory and powers. Therefore, it is not uncommon to see hens eating beside a particular cock. Hens will only get closer to a cock they feel will protect them from an attack whatsoever.

Chickens enjoy dust bath: There are times you would notice sand heaps in your garden, right? Your chickens are responsible for such an act. They enjoy digging the ground and making holes where they can rest. With this, they are certain of keeping their body temperatures normal, especially when the sun is too hot.

They are friendly: Contrary to what people think of, chickens are very friendly animals. This is why some individuals regard them as pets. Nonetheless, some chicken breeds are friendlier than others. So, before concluding that your chickens are not friendly, be certain to understand the breed of chicken on your poultry farm. Therefore, it is not uncommon to see chickens in nursery and other places because they are considered harmless.

The amount of feed your chickens consume determines their eggs' production: If you want your chicken to produce more eggs, feed them accordingly. About one dozen of eggs are produced after your chickens have consumed four pounds of feed. It is this quantity that helps them produce the number of eggs you desire.

Traditional breeds of chicken are becoming extinct: Many poultry farmers are trying to be economical with the feed they provide their chickens with. for this reason, they tend to favor hybrid chickens because they require less feed than the traditional breed of chickens. If this continues, it will not be strange to discover some breeds of chickens going into extinction over time.

Chickens speak in their language: While this seems to be impossible, it is actually true. Chickens communicate using their language. Research has it that chickens have at least about 30 sounds that they used for communicating. Interestingly, these sounds convey one thing or another. These sounds range from the need to raise an alarm, food, or to indicate an imposing danger. For instance, roosters will also make sounds to indicate the presence of foods to hens and also will make another sound to show hens of a particular nesting box.

How to speak the chicken language

Can one communicate with chickens? This sounds like an incredible task. But, it is possible. In this book, it has been stated that chickens have their language. If you must communicate with them, you need to understand what their sounds indicate and how to respond to the circumstance.

Chickens have different sounds for any situation that applies to them. Thus, when chickens come close to you, they make a particular sound, and this is their means of saying 'hello' to you. But, how do you know this, and what do you do next? In the same way, when you go close to eggs laid by a broody hen, she makes some sounds to indicate you should stay far away from her eggs as possible.

Sometimes, when you fail to do this, she uses her beak on you. Also, when there is any danger lurking around, she makes some noise to let you know of such. When chickens want to lay their eggs, they also announce it. But, if you do not know of this sound, you don't even know what to do. Even after laying the eggs, the chicken will still indicate that she had laid her eggs successfully. Sometimes, other hens would join her in celebrating the production of the egg.

If another hen has occupied her nesting box, she would always indicate that she wants to make use of the box so that the other hen would make room for her. It is evident that chicken language can be very tasking to learn, but it is achievable with conscious effort. Thus, it is important you get familiar with the differences in the languages chicken speak so that you would be able to do what is necessary at the right time.

To effectively communicate with chickens, you need to listen attentively to them. When you pay close attention to them when they communicate with each other, you would know the various sounds they make indicate. After listening to them, make attempts to speak back to them. This gesture will strengthen the bond you have with them and train them to listen and act towards simple commands that you would give to them.

The ways you can employ to communicate to your chickens are:

Mimic them: To communicate with your chickens, ensure that you imitate them at all times. You can start by listening to the way a mother hen calls her chicks. Try to find out what the sound means. Perhaps, she has found a new feeding place, and she wants them to come and eat what she has seen. The sound she makes sounds more like "Kruk Kruk." When she makes this sound, it is necessary that you understand what she has said and also respond to her accordingly.

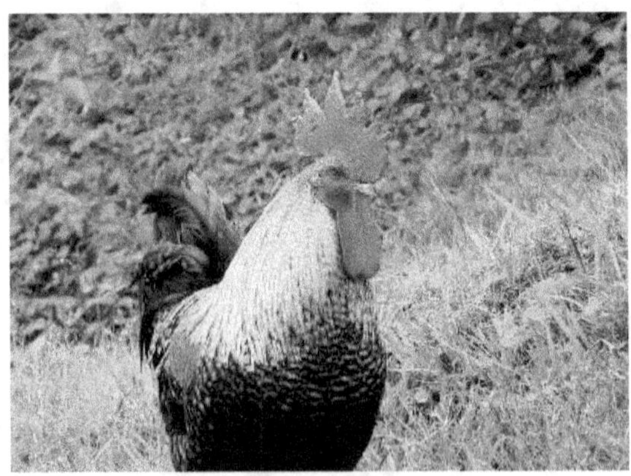

Pay attention to distress calls: When your chicken goes through any form of distress, she will squeak loud. It is your responsibility to respond to her at such times. Do not be in a hurry to dismiss the sounds she makes as irrelevant. Instead, understand that your chickens are probably telling you something that would be of interest to you. If it happens, you are the one who captured the chicken, and it makes a noise, be careful so that other chickens would not attack you for trying to take their friend away. Peradventure, you notice your chick are the one making noise, quickly go out and discover what is wrong with them. There could be chances that they are under some sort of threat.

Train them accordingly: If you want the best from your chickens, train them! Communicating with them is much easier when you use a particular word for them repeatedly. When they get familiar with the word you are using on them, it will be easier for you to communicate with them. This implies for every action that you want to carry out that is related to them, you should make use of a specific word. In communicating with your chicken, you can also make use of a bell as a means of training them. Perhaps, you want them to come to get their feed; you can use a bell to call them to the desired location. With time, whenever they hear the sound of the bell, they will associate it with food. In that way, you are making them interpret the bell's sound to make time to eat. If you do this successfully, you have trained them to communicate with you effectively.

CHAPTER NINE
LANDSCAPE GARDENING WITH CHICKENS

Beautifying your chicken environment with flowers would have them feeling special and excited. It is a fantastic way to spread the love you have in your heart for them. Fortunately, there are no special skills required to make this possible. All that you need is your sense of imagination and creativity. Moreover, what counts the most is your motive for wanting to do such. In doing this, you need to take extra care so that you don't plant toxic plants that can negatively affect your chickens. The only issue that may border you is to know the right type of plants to use when beautifying your chicken environment. It is also important to note that your chickens may likely consume your plants, but that shouldn't be too much of a problem for you.

The secret to a beautiful chicken yard

There are many ways to keep your chicken yard beautiful and make it attractive to everyone that comes across it. There is a lot more to be done in your chicken yard rather than pile up feeders and beddings. Remember that it is "home" for your chickens, and as such, you ought to give it every feel of a home, which implies making it look beautiful to them. There are a host of things that you can use in making your chicken yard look good. They include:

Flowers/plants: These include both edible and non-edible ones. It is good to have a handful of flowers/plants in your chicken yard. Asides from the fact that it makes their habitat look nice, it also produces a pleasant fragrance. Examples of flowers that can be added to the chicken yard are rose flowers, sunflower, violets, Iris, etc.

The use of shrubs: These also appeal to the eyes and give them a feeling of nature. Your chickens would love nothing more than being close to nature. So, this is a good idea to introduce in your chicken yard. Lavender, Juniper, and wormwood are good examples of shrubs you need to have in your chicken yard.

Be creative: It is your responsibility to make your chicken yard look as beautiful as you want it to be. Thus, you are permitted to use your senses and imagination to give the chicken yard a personal touch. This presupposes that you can choose paint colors of your choice. You can also improvise to get the right type of structural elements you need in your chicken yard. The use of wire mesh is not a bad idea to introduce into your chicken yard. It also serves other purposes asides from aesthetic use only.

Put up a name sign: You may not have thought about it before now, but giving your chicken yard a name makes it feel more like home. Moreover, always be guided with the thought that your chicken yard is their habitat. The same way you may want to put up a sign in front of your own house, they deserve the same.

Also, making your chicken yard beautiful comes with so many benefits. Some of these benefits stem from the fact that your chickens are protected from the grasp of predators. This is so because predators may experience difficulty in seeing your chickens in their coop. Furthermore, the plants that you plant in the chicken yard would also attract various types of insects, and your chickens would gladly feed on these nutritious insects. Also, your chickens will make use of the shade that the tree provides to keep themselves warm. You must agree that there would be times when the weather would be too hot for your chickens. The shades of the tree will be a good source for them to stay away from the heat temperature.

Chicks, Tricks and Tips

Chicks are cute and friendly, and as such, they require special care and attention to ensure they are protected from harm and harsh weather conditions that may affect their well-being.

The first thing to do before getting your chicks from the hatchery is to set up their brooder. A brooder is a place where the chicks would be made to rest. In constructing the brooder, certain items like a heat lamp, netting, cardboard box/wood box, feeders, thermometer, and other necessary items ensure their comfort. In setting up their brooder, get a good room where you can place the cardboard box/wood box. Ensure you lay some old newspapers in the bottom of the box and pour some wood chips into it.

Then, keep your thermometer in the box and fill the feeders and waterers with food and water, respectively. After doing this, put your heat lamp into the box and go and get your chicks.

A mix of some old-time wisdom and modern methods

Since time immemorial, poultry farmers had always devised a means of rearing chickens for either egg or meat production. These methods that those framers employed were sufficient to produce healthy and happy chickens. Today, the agricultural world has taken a different turn due to the advent of technological development and creative ideas. Nonetheless, both methods are still necessary for ensuring that poultry framers get the very best from their flocks. Some of the methods are:

The free-range poultry farming method:

In this poultry farming method, the chickens are allowed to roam around freely for a certain period. Thus, the poultry farmers do not use strict methods of raising the chickens. During the daytime, chickens would freely walk around their habitat, but at night, they would retire to their coop to be safe from the reach of predators. This method's effectiveness was dependent on certain variables such as a good location, appropriate drainage system, and good ventilation. Also, the poultry farmers also lookout for the right type of environment with a minimal number of predators. While this method is advantageous in that the chicken's droppings could serve as manure to make plants and flowers look healthy, it also has some disadvantages. Some of the disadvantages stem from the fact that the chickens are usually exposed to harsh weather conditions such as heat and cold. Also, the chickens may be exposed to predatory threats and diseases of all sorts.

The organic method of poultry farming: There are huge similarities between the free-range poultry farming method and the organic poultry framing difference. But, what makes them appear different is that the chickens are raised in large quantities for the free-range system, but in the organic method, the chickens are raised in smaller numbers.

Yarding poultry farming method: In this method, the farmer does not raise only chickens alone. He chooses a particular location and raises both poultry and cattle together. In this system, the cows and chickens are permitted to roam around freely in a confined space. They may not necessarily share a sleeping house, but they are allowed to move around their environment.

The battery cage poultry farming method: This is a common means of raising chickens in poultry farming. The use of small battery cages characterizes this method, usually made up of materials like mesh or metal. In each cell, about three or five chickens are kept. These battery cages possess wire mesh and collector layers that allow faeces and eggs to be properly collected without creating too much mess. In this method, feeding the chickens is very easy as the cage possesses a bisected metal where their food is kept and another space where water is made available to them. Without a doubt, this method comes with its advantages and disadvantages, but it is regarded as the most modern poultry farming method.

Husbandry practices

What does animal husbandry mean?

Animal husbandry is simply all animal welfare-related activities centered on the development and general wellbeing of animals and livestock. With this definition, it is very obvious that every poultry farmer is expected to take proper care of their chickens by making provision for all of their feeding, housing and developmental needs.

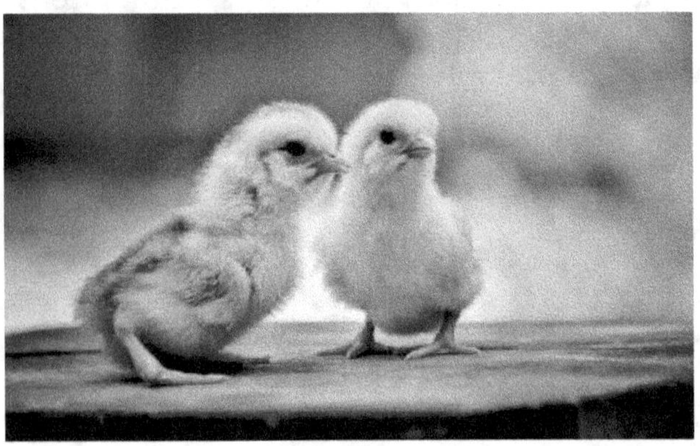

Good husbandry practices for chickens

Some good husbandry practices for chickens that all poultry farmers must take cognizance of are:

Keep harmful animals away: There are some animals whose presence would affect the well-being of your chickens. This is only because they are predators, and they feed on your chickens and their produce. Examples of such animals are rats, wild birds, and rats. As a rule, ensure that your chicken coop and run are well-constructed to hinder the presence of these destructive animals. Unfortunately, rats/mice are very known to transmit diseases. So, when they go into your chicken coop or run, they will most likely infect them with the diseases they carry.

On the other hand, wild birds transmit bird flu to your chickens. Thus, when the saliva or droppings of an infected wild bird comes in contact with your chicken, be certain that they have contracted bird flu. Do you want to avoid this? Keep them away from rats/mice and wild birds.

Store grains properly: Rats can perceive the smell of food from a very long distance. So, when you store grains in your chicken coop or close to their environment, it is evident you are calling rats to a feast. Guess what? They would come fully prepared to attack your chickens and the grains as well. To protect your grain, store them in metal containers that have a cover lid. With this, the grains will be kept far away from their reach and smell.

Isolate new chickens: The only way to stay safe as a poultry farmer is to favor healthy husbandry practices. This implies that when you purchase new chickens that you keep them separate from the older ones. It is not always easy to detect that a chicken is ill. Therefore, the only way to make sure that the new additions would not affect the other chickens' health in the coop is to keep them in a separate place for two weeks. If they do not show any signs or symptoms of being ill/sick at the end of two weeks, you can comfortably introduce them to the chicken coop.

Give them clean water: Of course, their health should be of paramount importance to you. This is because when your chickens are healthy, you are certain of making good profits off them and enjoying their productivity as well. While food is important to them, chickens can survive for a while without food. But, their survival in those times depends on the availability of clean water for them to drink. Chickens can drink up any type of water, but if you want to prevent the chances of getting infected with a disease, you should provide them with clean water.

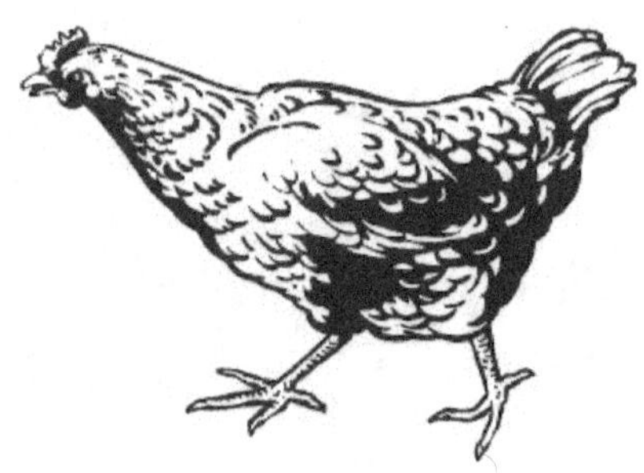

Maintain their coop: It is necessary to reiterate that the coop is their habitat. Thus, in the same way, you respect your homes and keep it clean, do the same for your chicken coop. When their coop is littered with droppings, this attracts flies. What about flies? They will infect your chickens' food and water, which would result in various forms of diseases. Flies breed easily, and unfortunately, a dirty chicken coop is a good breeding ground for flies. Avoid having wet food and beddings in the coop, as this is a great way to attract flies into the coop.

Feed them with a moderate amount of treats: Even in loving your chickens, there needs to be moderation! If you want to shower them with excessive love and feed them with various treats, it may cause more harm than good. In feeding your chicken with treats, moderation is key.

When you give them treats in moderation, it saves them the pain associated with having liver issues. It also saves you some losses which you may incur as a result of their illness. If treats must be offered to chickens, it needs to be healthy treats that would not affect their health in any way.

Figure out planting gardens in the coop

Chicken and gardens walk hand-in-hand. Why? Gardens thrive on the abundance of manure to help them blossom and look attractive. On the other hand, chickens are very significant in providing manure that is necessary for the survival and development of gardens. Now, it is obvious that chickens play a crucial role in the development of your garden; it is necessary to get the right type of plants to grow in your garden. While chickens would always enjoy tilling the ground in search of food and worm to eat, it is necessary to plant the right type of plants so that their lives don't become affected.

The presence of chicken amongst your plants would mean that you are prepared to accept all that comes with them being on your farm. This means that you would tolerate many of their foraging habits like dust bathing, eating up new seedlings, and destroying growing plants in your garden. This requires choosing an appropriate place to plant your flowers so that chickens do not ruin their leaves and stem. So, if you want your plants to grow healthy and blossom well, keep your chickens away from the garden until the plants are properly grown.

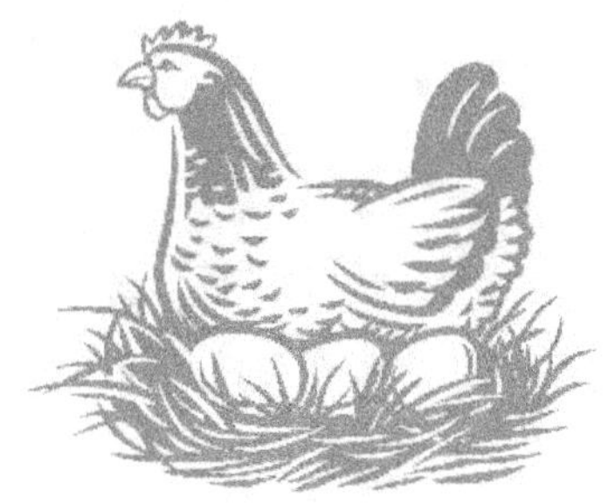

Construct a fence around your chicken coop when you plant flowers in them. This would keep away destructive predators that may also want to cause some harm to the plants that you have grown in the chicken environment. You can also decide to keep a separate run for your chickens or favor the idea of a raised bed. With this, there will be minimal damage that the chickens can cause to the plants. Some of the types of plants that can be planted around the chicken coop are herbs, amaranth, white clover, sunflowers, garlic, cucumbers, corn, dandelions, and leafy greens.

CHAPTER TEN
PET THERAPY

What is pet therapy?

Therapy animals are trained to be sociable and provide some sort of comfort to their owners. These animals are essential in helping their owners, and other individuals get relief from the stress that goes on around them. Interestingly, they are a good way to keep your children and other younger one's company. That is, these animals make good companions.

The uses of therapy animals range from one environment to the other. They play significant roles in the hospital. In the hospital, therapy animals are used during counseling sessions to help patients become relaxed and comfortable. The beauty of therapy animals is that their presence in the hospital environment is a good way of cheering individuals.

In the home, animal therapy benefits children immensely. In families with children and special needs or disabilities, animal therapy is very beneficial and helps such a child tremendously. Also, when there is a child who struggles with anger issues and other unpleasant behavior forms, animal therapy can help control such negative actions. Why? In handling pets or animals, one requires patience. So, when a child with anger issues wants to fasten a pet's collar, such a child is forced to be patient and disregard every form of anger. There are even programs where certain animals like dogs are used to teach children how to read properly.

These animals are also used in the courtroom. Suppose there is a situation where an individual is finding it difficult to talk about their trauma or come face to face with perpetrators of evil. In that case, therapy animals are used to help such individuals feel at ease to talk about their trauma.

Types of therapy animals

Dogs: This is regarded to be man's best friend and companion. This is simply because this animal helps humans to be comfortable and relaxed. Therefore, it is not strange to see them at workplaces, malls, and even grocery places. They are friendly and completely harmless because they have been trained in that manner.

Cats: Cats are preferred by individuals that are intimidated by the presence of dogs. They look nicer than dogs and gentle. The only difference between using cats to dogs as a therapy animal is that there are certain tasks that dogs are trained to perform that cats cannot, and this is especially true in medical situations. But, they are good at checking up on patients and snuggling. Also, they are beneficial when it comes to helping older ones survive dementia.

Horses: These animals are relatively large, and taking care of them requires that one demonstrates an enviable level of patience. Thus, this therapy animal is the best animal to help individuals with attitudinal problems such as anger, learning disabilities, etc.

Birds: These animals can speak like humans, especially parrots. Parrots are used in various homes as a therapy animal. They can easily communicate if their owners train them properly. Thus, they are fascinating to watch and can be a great way of relieving stress. They also possess an enviable level of empathy and are good for emotional support.

Chicken Therapy

Less country chicken coop and more pet chicken?

According to an estimate reported by the Los Angeles Times, chickens in the United States will become the new family doggie. More than 1% of American families own a chicken. By the end of 2019, urban chicken houses will have increased by 400%. And in France, the 50% increase in chicks and chickens' sales among city dwellers had already aroused curiosity in 2011.

Hens can be affectionate and funny. They have rules and social hierarchies that they can transfer into their relationship with other species, such as humans.

Usually, for hens living with humans, the human being provides the food, and a relationship may be established for which we become the 'alpha hen'. Hens show the behavior of affiliation and rapprochement with humans as well.

The chickens could keep you company for a long time. They can live between five and eleven years, depending on the breed and the living and feeding conditions, which greatly influence longevity. An example: a laying hen that is born and lives in a healthy environment, outdoors and with a good diet can live eight or ten years, unlike a laying hen raised in a cage in a shed, which survives an average of three years.

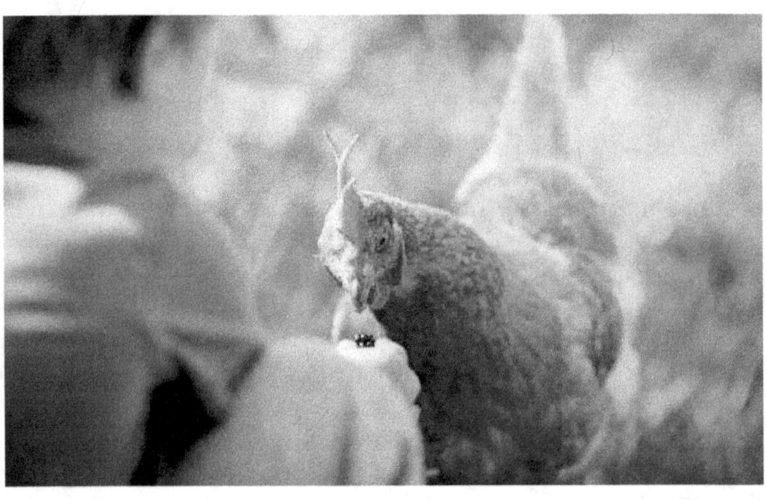

Autism and Therapy Chickens

From a study on the benefits of the farm environment, including animals, for autistic children. Studies have shown the calming power of hens on autistic children.

Keeping chickens and a chicken coop is also being praised as therapeutic for children on the autism spectrum. Families who keep chickens are getting their children with autism involved in feeding and caring for the chickens, promoting self-help and independent living skills. The chickens serve as a conversation starter for children who are shy and limited socially, thereby helping to improve their social skills with peers and adults. The children feel safe and open around the chickens and are able to play with them while playing with other children is often difficult. This increases the child's play skills.

To have hens-pets, it is not obligatory to have very large spaces, but: a green handkerchief where they can be raked, a shelter for the rain and that can protect them from possible predators, the earth where to dig in search of worms and where to make the "earth baths" - which serve to eliminate and prevent the presence of parasites.

How therapy animals are used as education for kids

Education is an all-encompassing word that requires instilling the right skills and attitudes into an individual. Therefore, education is not limited to the classroom environment alone. There are various skills and attitudes that children need to equip themselves with so that they can become valuable and instrumental to societal development.

Unfortunately, there are a couple of factors that mitigate children's ability to be properly educated to handle life challenges and issues. Some of these factors are hereditary and social. Whilst their parents and caregivers may have exhausted all tricks and ideas in their possession to make the child change for the better, a good method that can be employed is the use of animal therapy.

It is almost difficult to come across a child that does not admire animals. It may not necessarily be dogs, cats, or birds. But, there would be a certain type of animal the child fancies. Thus, if parents or caregivers must use animal therapy to educate their children, they must identify the type of animal the child admires. With this knowledge, it is easier to record results with the use of animal therapy.

Children who experience difficulty in showing empathy towards others can be corrected with the use of animal therapy. How? The parents and caregivers of such children can teach them to show care to the animals. When they do this, they tend to put themselves in the position of the animals and feel an understanding of the pain the animal goes through. In this way, such a change is introduced to being empathic to the plights of others. Even in doing this, the children are taught to have a sense of responsibility. Caring for animals requires a lot, and when children are taught in this manner, it helps them develop the right mindset and attitude towards life.

In animal therapy, as a means of educating children, the children are also made to understand patience. Children who may not be able to teach others would be taught how to teach their favorite animals new skills. As time progresses and the child begins to notice that the animal is adjusting to all that it is being taught, that child's self-esteem increases drastically. The child would begin to appreciate him/herself the more, especially after seeing how much positive he had with the animal. Thus, animal therapy is a good way to help children gain self-confidence.

This education technique also helps children to gain trust. In the course of the therapy, the child will begin to share a bond with the animal. By so doing, he becomes relaxed and slowly begins to trust the animal. This same attitude is also used to communicate effectively and build trust with others around him/her. Also, children learn how to give and receive unconditional love during animal therapy. This also makes them become more independent and require less assistance in getting things around them done.

Samantha Martines

CONCLUSION

Poultry farming is an admirable aspect of agricultural activities. A common part of poultry farming is raising chickens. Raising chickens is an enjoyable task but can also be very demanding. This is why it is necessary to delve into poultry farming with the right mindset, purpose, and attitude.

Inasmuch as poultry farming appears quite easy to individuals, it requires an in-depth understanding of what the practice entails. Failure to abide by the trade's necessary know-how can lead to failure even before the business or activity gets to the maturity stage. Budding poultry farmers must realize that poultry farming takes place even before the new chicks are hatched. This is so because they are expected to have addressed all the necessary levels of the activity before even bringing the chick home.

It is no news that chickens are very fragile animals, and as such, they require a lot of care and attention. Thus, there are many factors to consider in poultry farming for it to turn out a success. In raising chickens, poultry farmers must identify threats to the success of the activity and keep them at bay. In addition, adequate research is required to make the right choice of chicken breeds. For your chickens to remain healthy and happy, they must be fed with the right amount of feed, water, light, and medication. These animals are susceptible to various diseases. So, to avert circumstances where you record losses, it is important to pay attention to your chickens' health needs.

Interestingly, chickens also provide therapeutic benefits to their owners. They are fascinating creatures to watch and can be a good way to relieve stress and anxiety. More so, children can use these animals to learn about accepting responsibilities and other healthy manners.